A Field Guide for Activating the Learner

A Field Guide for Activating the Learner

Using the Learner's Brain Model

Dr. Mario C. Barbiere

ROWMAN & LITTLEFIELD
Lanham • Boulder • New York • London

Published by Rowman & Littlefield
An imprint of The Rowman & Littlefield Publishing Group, Inc.
4501 Forbes Boulevard, Suite 200, Lanham, Maryland 20706
www.rowman.com

Unit A, Whitacre Mews, 26-34 Stannary Street, London SE11 4AB

Copyright © 2018 by Mario C. Barbiere

All rights reserved. No part of this book may be reproduced in any form or by any electronic or mechanical means, including information storage and retrieval systems, without written permission from the publisher, except by a reviewer who may quote passages in a review.

British Library Cataloguing in Publication Information Available

Library of Congress Cataloging-in-Publication Data

Names: Barbiere, Mario C., author.
Title: A field guide for activating the learner : using the learner's brain model/ Mario C. Barbiere.
Description: Lanham, Maryland : Rowman & Littlefield, [2018] | Includes bibliographical references.
Identifiers: LCCN 2018010321 (print) | LCCN 2018026717 (ebook) | ISBN 9781475841237 (Electronic) | ISBN 9781475841213 (cloth : alk. paper) | ISBN 9781475841220 (pbk. : alk. paper)
Subjects: LCSH: Learning, Psychology of. | Learning--Physiological aspects. | Brain research
Classification: LCC LB1060 (ebook) | LCC LB1060 .B3725 2018 (print) | DDC 370.15/23--dc23
LC record available at https://lccn.loc.gov/2018010321

To Kermit, Jim and Mairin, Kaleb, Kaia;
Chris; Mike and Jackie; Matt, Sophie.

You give life meaning

Contents

Foreword	ix
Preface	xi
Acknowledgments	xiii
Introduction	1
1 Informational Stage: Lesson Delivery (Input Stage of Learner's Brain Model)	5
2 Middle Stage of Learner's Brain Model: Assessments	27
3 Closing Stage of Learner's Brain Model: Consolidation for Closure	53
4 Lesson Design: Reflection	67
5 Sample Lesson Plan: Putting It All Together	83
Appendix A Classroom Environment	101
Appendix B Differentiating Instruction	103
Appendix C Objective DSL Indicators	107
Appendix D Objective DSL Checklist	109
Appendix E Student Engagement	111
Appendix F Student Interviewing	113
Appendix G Use of Data	115
About the Author	117

Foreword

Teaching is rocket science. If it were not, merely attending school would produce students who are successful learners. It would produce students who were fully engaged in learning tasks in this age of technology. It would be the great equalizer that would ensure the civil right of quality education for all whom we are entrusted to teach. University schools of education would produce career educators who would be prepared to teach all learners.

Many years ago—too many to count—I became a teacher. I wanted to be the best possible teacher I could be and I quickly learned that I needed deeper knowledge of the science of teaching to address the diverse, compelling, and complicated intellectual, social, emotional, and physical needs of the students in front of me. Fortunately, I decided to go on a journey to become the "best possible teacher" I could be. It became clear that ensuring high-quality student outcomes was linked to high-quality teaching practices. And the foundation of that practice is the designing of high-quality lessons and knowing how students learn.

As promotional opportunities allowed me to move into the role of school principal, I was introduced to protocols that I could use to improve my teachers' instructional practices, collectively and collaboratively. Moreover, I was introduced to ways to use these protocols to support my growth as coach and mentor to each teacher. No matter how experienced the teacher, I found that one's greatest success as an educator occurs when one understands and plans for the learner. My faculty and I committed to working collaboratively to become the best teachers we could be. The protocols we used produced high-achievement outcomes for students during my 16 years as a principal.

As time would have it, my journey expanded to a role as a central office administrator. I am a strong advocate for assessing student learning by walking the classrooms that have been skillfully planned for the learner. Believe it or not, prepared classrooms are the teacher's most powerful tool and aid in the classroom. When the teacher's lesson is over, the students must have a classroom that continues to "teach" the lesson. The Walk Through Protocols are formative tools that go beyond the formal teacher observations of today: They are the building tools of the skilled teacher.

It was during this stage of my educational journey that I met Dr. Mario Barbiere during the phase in my career when I served as coach and mentor to principals. Our team of Turnaround Officers had combined experience of over 200 educator years.

Dr. Barbiere not only had the highest number of years of experience, he brought the wisdom and understanding in ways we could share our expertise. He understood we were not there to critique but to guide, collaborate, and urge these new leaders toward more efficient and effective practices—to the rocket science of education.

We talked and planned; we walked classrooms and discussed; we formed a dynamic team with a common vision of what instructional practices were important and how we could reproduce them in the leaders in our care. In the schools he coached, outstanding progress was made—achievement rose from 39% to 86% in less than three years, moving closer to 90/90/90 school improvement.

Dr. Barbiere took these discussions to another level, however. He brought years of research on brain learning theory, with years and years of experience to develop excellent tools for use by educators. His turned the rubrics into teaching tools for high-quality classrooms. He helped teachers understand their role to develop self-regulated learners. Coupled with intentional practices such as lesson design, engagement, and learning environments, he developed rubrics that could calibrate teaching practices across classrooms and schools.

The field guide that you are about to read will outline the essential elements and components of high-quality lessons—designing them purposefully and intentionally to optimize student learning. In essence, Dr. Barbiere's text provides the "science" of designing effective lessons to produce positive outcomes for student learning. This is what teachers labor to do. Now there are tools to help with that intentional plan to be successful. And that is what makes teaching rocket science.

Gayle W. Griffin, PhD
Educational Consultant
Seton Hall University–Academy of Urban School Transformation

Preface

As an educational practitioner who has worked closely with Dr. Barbiere for the past few years in closing the achievement gap in my school, I am excited to learn about this new text and the research base for which it is rooted.

What is different about Dr. Barbiere's approach is that he uses a combination of brain-based learning and self-regulation of learning to help guide learners through practical approaches that educators can employ immediately in their classrooms. What's more, Dr. Barbiere stands behind his espoused practices: He is in classrooms every day and has the benefit of having observed and implemented his tools in literally hundreds of classrooms in all socioeconomic and demographic populaces.

Dr. Barbiere shares practical tools and strategies for the educator to employ. More significant is that these practices help the learner to self-motivate, reflecting actively on their own learning and using these strategies to monitor their own progress. This is an empowering and important strategy for learners, especially those with learning and/or demographic disadvantages.

I endorse this text with full confidence that once the reader utilizes any or all of the research-based strategies discussed, you will see immediate differences in your classroom, school, or district, as I have in my own, thanks to the guidance and measurable methods provided within the text.

Dr. Michael Gaskell, Principal
East Brunswick Public Schools

Acknowledgments

Teaching is a dynamic profession, as it is an art as well as a science. I have used the feedback from teachers who have crafted their art in developing the rubrics. I used the research from the science of teaching for empirical data to support the rubrics. Using suggestions from teachers and research about the science of teaching, I was able to create worksheets and activities for teachers, administrators, parents, or students to use for promoting metacognition and self-regulation based on theory and practice.

The rubrics that were developed were field tested and I appreciate and acknowledge the input I received from my colleagues including Mike Vignola, Andrew White, Sam Garrison, Dr. Gayle Griffin, Dr. Scott Taylor, Bill Andersen, Sheila Wegryn, Neyda Evans, Frank Zalocki, Dr. Jo Ann Berkley, Dr. Fran Borkes, John Neisz, Scott LoRocca, Jane Wiatr, Dr. Pat Mitchell, Dr. Mike Gaskell, Ras Baraka, and countless other administrators and teachers. I appreciate your feedback and support.

I also appreciate and acknowledge the support my extended family has provided throughout this process. Thanks John and Pat, Jim and Diane, Janice and Mark, Carol and Mark.

A very special acknowledgement goes to educators everywhere who go to work every day to help students realize their dreams. Teaching is indeed a noble profession. As educators, you bring hope and that is what makes the profession rewarding.

Thank you Carlie Wall and Tom Koerner as well as Rowman & Littlefield for making my dream become a reality.

To the administrators who dare to dream and believe that they make a difference: Never give up the dream as parents and students trust us and believe in us. Our job is to make the dreams come true.

Introduction

I never thought I would be interested in writing a field guide about brain research and lesson delivery. After all, my doctorate was on brain research and lesson design so I did spend years researching the topic. It was truly fascinating to understand how information is processed in the brain and what teachers can do to ensure that the information goes from short-term memory to long-term memory.

Since my three sons and daughter-in-law are educators, I see the amount of time they spend on lesson plans. I also see how frustrated they get when students are not "getting it." That prompted me into thinking: Teaching is an art as well as a science, and having spent years studying brain research and lesson design, I recognize that there are strategies that can be employed to engage the learner. The challenge was on! I could draw upon practical knowledge and brain research theory to provide a meaningful field guide.

Having worked in education as an administrator supervising teachers, I was aware of what effective instruction looks like. More importantly, after years of doing coaching walks and walk-throughs, I did not meet a teacher who was not willing to learn or improve their pedagogy. Teachers were eager for feedback and were receptive to peer coaching so I reasoned that teachers would be receptive to a field guide with activities and rubrics that they can use.

My experience in working with teachers was varied, but I particularly enjoyed working with teachers involved in school turnaround. I had been assigned as a network turnaround officer to two low-performing schools in New Jersey. I had the opportunity to work with teachers who were eager to hone their craft and ensure that their students would be successful. That position was part of a School Improvement Grant (SIG), which was subsidize by Race to the Top money. As the federal funds started to shrink, New Jersey had submitted a waiver from the No Child Left Behind requirements. The plan was to build upon the successes of the network turnaround officers and provide resources, via regional achievement centers for low-performing schools or schools with an achievement gap.

New Jersey's waiver from No Child Left Behind sought to establish six regional achievement centers that would work with schools that had been identified as low-performing or schools that had a 43.5 percent achievement gap between the highest-performing subgroup and the average of the two lowest performing subgroups. As executive director for Regional Achievement Center 5, I had the opportunity to visit the identified low-performing schools and/or schools identified as having an achievement gap. I would work with teachers and they would ask for suggestions for improvement. I decided that I would spend my weekends continuing my research that I had started with my doctoral dissertation to see what rubrics and/or strategies I could develop that would be useful for teachers to use in the classroom.

My passion grew as I was spending my time on the weekends expanding the research I had done for my doctoral studies. I would develop rubrics and strategies that could be used in the classroom for teachers based on brain research and how the learner learns. The task was to understand the nature of the learner and not try to "fix" teachers.

My wife gave me encouragement and provided a focus. As a former teacher she would question me and ask what evidence I had. She truly was my greatest supporter and my most critical eye, forcing me to use empirical research in the work. After seven years of doing research, working at night or on the weekends, I developed two textbooks: *Setting the Stage: Delivering the Plan Using the Learner's Brain Model* and *Activating the Learner's Brain Using the Learner's Brain Model* and two field guides to support the textbooks or to serve as stand-alone guides.

This field guide begins with lesson delivery. Teachers interested in developing lesson plans are asked to consult the text *Setting the Stage: Teaching to the Learner's Brain* or *Field Guide for Setting the Stage: Delivering the Plan by Using the Learner's Brain Model* that addresses the planning stage of instruction. This field guide addresses the instructional phase by providing strategies and activities related to teacher-directed instruction, student-directed instruction, independent work, small group activities and/or cooperative activities.

A popular technique for instructional delivery is to use a "gradual release" strategy of "I do" (the teacher providing instruction); "we do" (teacher and student(s) do activities); and "you do" (the student does the work). The strategies involved in gradual release start with large group instruction that is teacher directed. The "we do" phase involves small group work that includes many "cooperative activities" that can be done to engage students.

Based on information the teacher receives during the instructional process, the next question is how will the teacher use the information and data obtained during the instructional process to plan subsequent lessons?

Chapter 2 will focus on how to use assessments, ways to develop assessments and assessment activities, which will ensure that student progress is monitored. By using formative and summative assessments and using data to drive instruction, assessments provide data for future lesson planning.

The focus of the chapter is on analyzing data so the teacher is not "data rich" and "analysis poor." The following probing questions will be answered: How will the information from the assessments be used? How will my assessments be tied to standards? How will I know if my assessments provide data to me about my students and if they are learning throughout the lesson? What are assessment activities I can use that incorporate different learning modalities?

A guiding question is: Are tests and assessments our friend or our foe? They can be our foe if a student takes a test, does poorly, and becomes discouraged, frustrated, or upset. However, tests and assessments can be our friend if the teacher uses information, for example, checking for understanding or formative assessments for monitoring and adjusting the learning.

The assessment strategies are done throughout the instructional period to assess if the student knows or understands the material, thereby enabling the teacher to pace his or her lesson.

If the goal is to develop self-regulated related learners, it is the student who must engage in assessment to promote the process of regulation.

After the introductory chapter, which talks about instructional delivery, chapter 2 discusses assessment during the instructional delivery phase and provides assessments; the third chapter addresses the conclusion of the lesson or Consolidation for Closure.

Consolidation for Closure is a process whereby the learner will summarize what has been learned. Although closure is usually done at the end of a lesson, it can be done throughout the lesson. One strategy for closure is using Demonstrations of Student Learning (DSL).

This chapter addresses the following questions:

1. What is Consolidation for Closure?
2. When is Consolidation for Closure done?
3. How does Consolidation for Closure affect student learning?

Consolidation for Closure is a process whereby the learner will summarize what has been learned. The student had time to practice and rehearse what was taught and attach sense and meaning to the learning. The specific student talk and summary provides information to the teacher. Although closure is usually done at the end of a lesson, there are various other times it is effective.

Consolidation for Closure can start a lesson, be found in the middle of a lesson, and it can close a lesson, which is called terminal closure. It may be hard to imagine closure any place other than at the end of a lesson, but the true definition of closure, as it applies to teaching and lesson design is a review and summation of the subject matter presented before, during, or after a lesson is delivered.

The information that the teacher has gathered throughout the lesson and at the conclusion of the lesson when she does closure is critical as the teacher reflects on the data and uses it to plan for the next lesson. The field guide offers strategies for overt and covert closure and closure for visual, auditory, kinetic, and tactile preferred learners.

Reflection is an important phase for lesson design, instructional delivery, and professional growth. Although Students Learning Targets (objectives) were met, how does the teacher know the students learned what was intended for them to learn? What additional resources will the teacher need to further enhance the lesson? What would the teacher do differently next time? All of these questions are a few of the reflection questions that teachers can ask as they begin the planning process for subsequent lessons. The chapter on Reflection, chapter 4, also includes preplanning questions the teacher can use for the reflective process.

The final chapter, chapter 5, provides a sample lesson and breaks down components of the lesson. The sample lesson will provide insights to the reader on how the Learner's Brain Model can be applied. Even though each school district has their own requirement for writing lesson plans, there are basic elements for all lesson plan templates.

In the appendix I have provided rubrics that teachers can use to self-assess their instructional practice or to use for peer coaching. Administrators can also use the rubrics for professional development, grade level meetings, professional learning community meetings, or coaching teachers. Rubric are included for: classroom environment, differentiated instruction, objective and demonstration of student learning indicators, objective and demonstration of student learning checklist, student engagement, student interviews, and use of data.

I invite readers to use the material and provide feedback, comments, suggestions, or changes that can be made for improvement.

1

Informational Stage

Lesson Delivery (Input Stage of Learner's Brain Model)

FOCUS OF THE CHAPTER

The informational stage of the Learner's Brain Model, proposed by Dr. Barbiere, involves providing teacher-directed instruction, student-directed instruction, independent work, small group activities, and/or cooperative activities. Strategies for each phase of the Informational Stage will be provided.

INTRODUCTION

How does the Learner's Brain Model use right and left brain research for lesson design? Why lessons need the logical (left brain) and the global perspective (right brain) is important as educators move from the "informational" age to the "conceptual" age. How to plan lessons by applying information and concepts to real life problems. Additionally, how lessons can be planned using brain research and how the learner processes information so the lessons are more effective.

PROBING QUESTIONS

1. How do I plan a lesson using brain research about the nature of the learner?
2. What is gradual release?
3. Competency vs. performance?
4. How does the teacher pace the lesson?

Delivery of Instruction (Input)

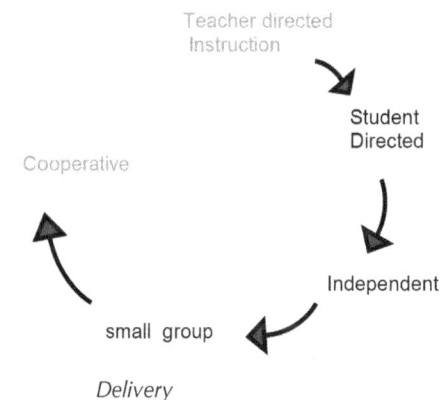

Activity Sheet for Informational Delivery Stage of the Learner's Brain Model

Using the model below, describe what you will do during each stage.

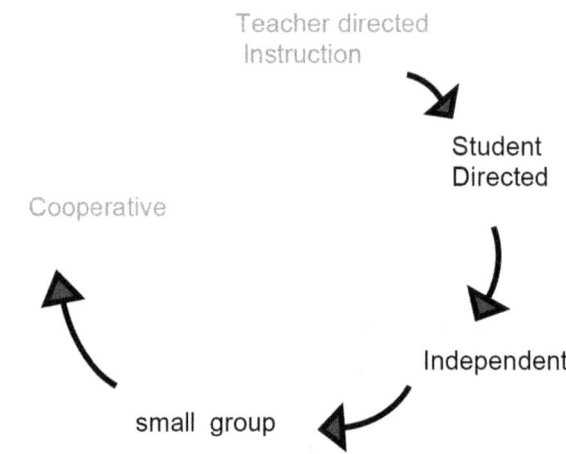

(Input Stage)

Teacher-directed stage I will

Independent stage I will

Small group stage I will

Cooperative stage I will

Reflection:

Reflective Questions for Engaging Students in Learning

> **Focus: The students are cognitively challenged and develop understanding of the concepts taught by what they are doing. The grouping of students, the activities and assignments planned, the instructional materials and resources selected, and the pacing of the lesson are critical components of the element.**

- Are all students cognitively involved in understanding important content? Are they actively participating and making genuine contributions to the effort?
- Student engagement is not the same as "busy" or "time on task." Mere activity is inadequate for cognitive engagement. Does the activity represent new learning, or intellectual, cognitive involvement?
- Is the material cognitively challenging for the student's level?
- Are a teacher's decisions about student grouping based on a number of considerations? Most important, does the type of instructional group reflect what a teacher is trying to accomplish so the grouping serves that purpose?
- Are instructional materials and resources suitable for the students and applicable to the instructional outcomes?
- Is there a recognizable beginning, middle, and end (closure)?

> **Look for: Students are "working" and not watching the teacher; high level of student thinking and activity; students are taking initiatives to modify or improve the lesson; there is a clear structure for the lesson with appropriate pacing.**

Since the curriculum standards will drive instructional delivery, it is important that teachers consider the following questions when planning for the instructional delivery phase. Planning and evaluating the lesson are important, therefore the most critical question will address how a teacher will determine the starting point of the lesson?

1. What do the students already know about the topic, so I can determine what content will be taught? (Content question)
2. What standards will I be addressing relative to the content? (Curriculum alignment to standards-based instruction)
3. What assessment information do I have that gives me the starting point for instructional planning? (Use of assessments to plan and differentiate instruction)
4. What can I expect my students to know by the end of the lesson? (Use of an Essential Question to establish long-term goal)
5. What do I expect my students to know at the end of the lesson? [Short-term goal for the development of the Student Learning Target (Objective)]
6. How will I present the information to activate student interest and promote readiness? (A Readiness Set is needed to establish an effective emotional climate)
7. What resources will be needed to meet the Student Learning Target objective? (Resources needed to implement the teaching process).
8. How will I know if the students understand the content? (Will I use checks for understanding/formative assessments and questions throughout the lesson?)
9. How will I close the lesson and gather information for planning subsequent lessons? (Consolidation for Closure activities)

Table 1.2. Lesson Planning Handout

Planning question: Content	Yes/No	Reflection
What do the students already know about the topic so I can determine what content will be taught?		Need to assess students' prior knowledge
What standards will I be addressing relative to the content?		Curriculum alignment to standards-based instruction
Planning questions Instructional delivery		Question to use to plan delivery
How will I present the information to activate student interest and promote readiness?		A Readiness Set is needed to establish an effective emotional climate
What assessment information do I have that gives me the starting point for instructional planning?		Use of assessments to plan and differentiate instruction
What do I *expect* my student to know at the end of the lesson?		Short-term goal for the development of the Student Learning Target (Objective)
What resources will be needed to accomplish meeting the objective?		Resources needed to implement the teaching process
Planning Questions Assessments		What assessments am I planning to use?
What *can* I expect my students to know by the end of the lesson?		Use of an Essential Question to establish a long-term goal
How will I know if the students understand the content?		Use of checks for understanding/formative assessments and questions
How will I close the lesson and gather information for planning subsequent lessons?		Consolidation for closure

Notes

Table 1.3. How Will the Teacher Know What the Students Already Know?

The answer to this question is *"pre-assessment."* The teacher will use a formative assessment. A formative assessment is the use of informal or formal testing materials which enables the teacher to gather data prior, during, or even after the learning process. The teacher records the information and modifies the curriculum so that the learning activities are differentiated and meet the cognitive needs of the student.
What formative assessments will I use during the lesson?
What data did I collect from the formative assessments?
How will I use the data for future lessons?
Reflection

Notes

INTERPRETING THE PRE-ASSESSMENTS

Interpretation of the pre-assessment will provide information to the teacher about what the students know. The information that is gained can be used as a starting point for instruction, since each student has a different starting point. Through focusing on formative assessment, teachers see that differentiation is not a single event to plan for but, rather, a process that occurs naturally when teachers set goals.

The theory behind the use of assessments for planning differentiation empowers teachers to learn about their student's needs and then leads the teacher into responding to these needs appropriately. The value of doing a formative assessment is that an effective formative assessment ensures instructional alignment among standards, objectives, and learning activities.

Normally, formative assessments are used throughout the lesson to collect data; however, the data collection process can also begin at the end of the previous lesson. The teacher will do an assessment (Consolidation for Closure activity) at the end of the lesson and the closure activity will provide information regarding what content and material should be developed for the subsequent lesson.

EXAMPLES OF ASSESSMENTS

A teacher chooses to use an "exit ticket" (tell me one thing you learned today or write down one thing that was confusing). The information or data collected by the teacher when the student answers the exit question will be critical in planning the next day's lesson. The use of an exit card or any other Consolidation for Closure activity addresses question number one: What does the student knows about the content? Based upon the student's answer on the exit ticket, the teacher may consider re-teaching aspects of the lesson or proceeding with a new lesson.

After the information from the Consolidation for Closure activity is reviewed by the teacher and student progress is assessed, then and only then, the teacher begins the process of developing lessons based on the new information. The teacher should decide what strategies will be useful for building success: large group instruction, small group instruction, independent practice, peer/buddy support.

Preassessment Chart

Preassessment

Interpretation

Next Step

Table 1.4. Activity for Planning Assessments

Standards to be assessed
Planned assessments
Why are the planned assessments the best assessments to use?
What were the results of the planned assessments?
Next steps

USING ASSESSMENTS FOR PLANNING INSTRUCTIONAL DELIVERY

The large group approach can be used to introduce the lesson, which is done in the pre-instructional phase. This approach captures everyone's attention and begins a process of activating prior knowledge, as well as helping the students see the big picture. After the teacher identifies the Student Learning Target (objective) and Essential Question to the class, a readiness activity is conducted. The Readiness Set will help focus the student's attention (the hook) and link the new knowledge with the prior knowledge (the connect).

SUGGESTIONS FOR INSTRUCTION

The teacher should remember that each lesson contains specific strategies that she will want to implement. These strategies are not lesson designs per se, but do reflect what the teacher needs to deliver and what the student objective is for each lesson. I will briefly list these items with a brief description in this workbook.

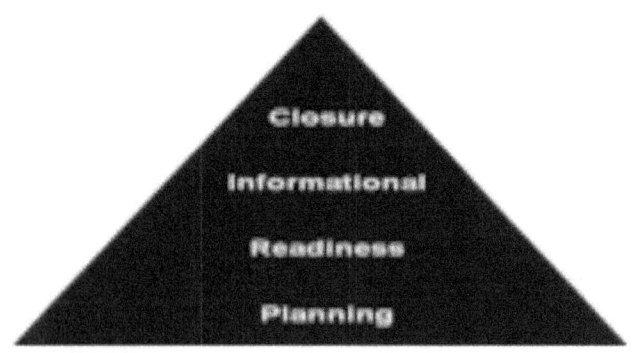

Learner's Brain Model

INSTRUCTIONAL INPUT FOR THE INFORMATIONAL STAGE

Instructional Input is the part of the lesson during which the teacher teaches the skills or provides the information to the student so the student can reach the predetermined Student Learning Target (Objective). One way for the teacher to help students self-regulate is for the teacher to model self-regulation strategies. Modeling is necessary because self-regulation strategies must be learned and practiced.

Modeling

Modeling is an important form of classroom support for learning. Students need to learn strategies and practice them in class so when they are at home or away from the classroom, they have strong foundational skills and can do the task independently. The key: Practice makes perfect, so one has to make sure that the practice is "correct" or perfect.

Input (Activities)

In planning input activities the teacher must have the information—standards, student background, materials needed, assessments needed, time allocations, and Consolidation for Closure before the planning can begin.

Table 1.5. What Formative Assessments Will I Use to Check for Understanding

What is the desired output? Knowing the end will help the teacher to plan skills to accomplish the desired result.
What will I do? What instructional activities will you use?
What do the students do? What engagement strategies will the students do?
How will the learning be measured? What assessment procedures will be used?

Table 1.6. Planning Chart

How will the teacher know that students are learning? Think about specific questions you can ask students in order to check for understanding to ask the questions in different ways.
What questions are planned to ask students to check for understanding?
What will students do to demonstrate that they understand what is being taught?
Going back to the Student Learning Target (Objectives), what activities will the teacher do to check whether each of those has been accomplished?

USING MULTIPLE PATHWAYS (INTELLIGENCES) FOR DEMONSTRATIONS OF STUDENT LEARNING (DSL)

The teacher can use Multiple Pathways to establish Demonstrations of Student Learning (DSL)

Linguistic: The student has the ability to use words effectively. These learners have highly developed auditory skills and often think in words. They like reading, playing word games, making up poetry or stories. They can be taught by encouraging them to say and see words, read books together. Tools include computers, games, multimedia, books, tape recorders, and lecture.

Logical–Mathematical: The student has capacity for reasoning and calculating. They are able to think conceptually, abstractly, and are able to see and explore patterns and relationships. They like to experiment, solve puzzles, and ask questions. They can be taught through logic games, investigations, and mysteries. They need to learn and form concepts before they can deal with details.

Musical: Student shows sensitivity to rhythm and sound. They love music, but they are also sensitive to sounds in their environments. They may study better with music in the background. They can be taught by turning lessons into lyrics, speaking rhythmically, and tapping out time. Tools include musical instruments, music, radio, DVD, CD-ROM, multimedia, computer.

Bodily–Kinesthetic: The student can use the body effectively, like a dancer or a surgeon. They have a keen sense of body awareness. They like movement, making things, touching. They communicate well through body language and can be taught through physical activity, hands-on learning, acting out, role playing. Tools include equipment and real objects.

Spatial–Visual: The student thinks in terms of physical space, as do architects and sailors. They are very aware of their environment. They like to draw, do jigsaw puzzles, read maps, or solve complex problems. They can be taught through drawings, verbal and physical imagery. Tools include models, graphics, charts, photographs, drawings, 3-D modeling, video, videoconferencing, television, multimedia, texts with pictures/charts/graphs.

Interpersonal: These students learn through interaction. They have many friends, empathy for others, street smarts. They can be taught through group activities, seminars, and dialogues. Tools include smart phones, audio conferencing, time and attention from the instructor, video conferencing, writing, computer conferencing, e-mail.

Intrapersonal: The student has understanding of their own interests and goals. These learners tend to shy away from others. They're in tune with their inner feelings; they have wisdom, intuition, and motivation, as well as a strong will, confidence, and opinions. They can be taught through independent study and introspection. Tools include books, creative materials, diaries, privacy, and time. They are the most independent of the learners.

Naturalist: Naturalistic is one of the most recent addition to Gardner's theory and has been met with some resistance. Individuals who are high in this type of intelligence are more in tune with nature and are often interested in nurturing, exploring the environment, and learning about other species. These individuals are said to be highly aware of even subtle changes to their environment.

As noted and shown in the graphic below, the informational stage involves providing teacher-directed instruction, student-directed instruction, independent work, small group activities, and/or cooperative activities. All of these strategies are part of the instructional delivery.

Instructional Delivery (Gradual release from teacher to student)

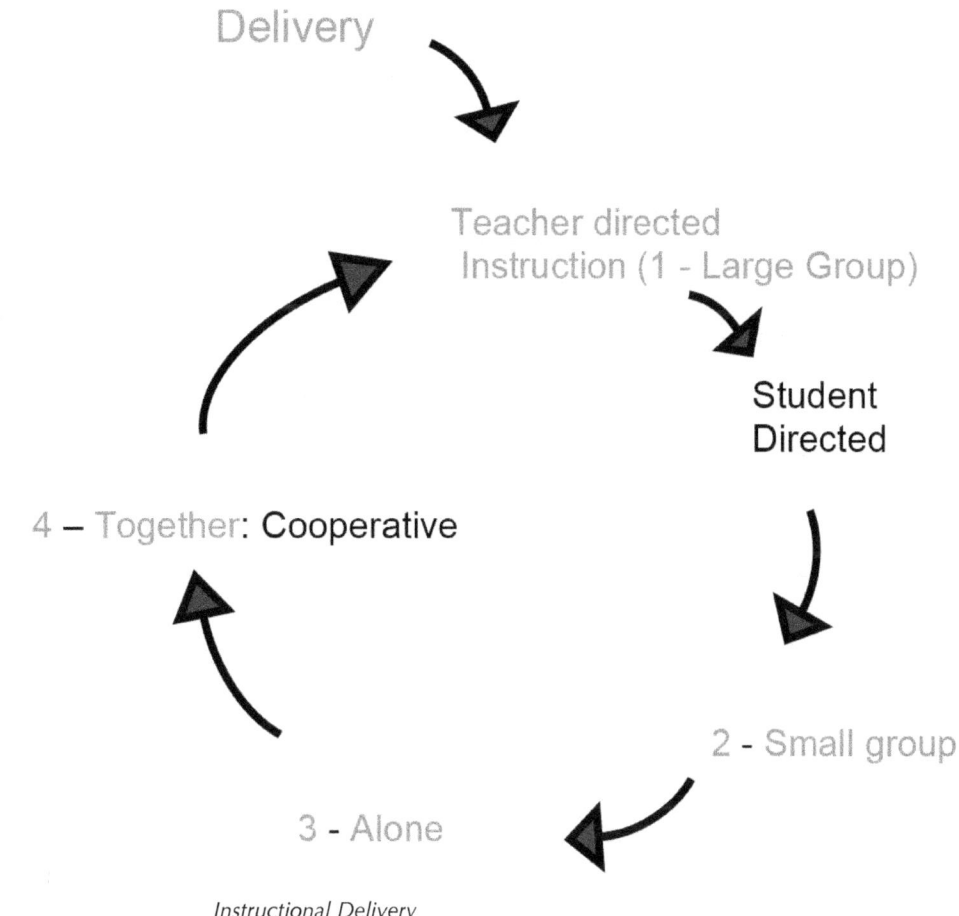

Instructional Delivery

PLANNING GUIDE

How will gradual releases occur?

How will I plan for students to all participate in small group activities?

How will I monitor small group activities?

What will I do with all the data I gather during the lesson?

Table 1.7. Demonstration of Student Learning (DSL) Planning Guide

Linguistic: They like reading, playing word games, making up poetry or stories. They can be taught by encouraging them to say and see words, read books together. Tools include computers, games, multimedia, books, tape recorders, and lecture. *DSL:*
Logical—Mathematical: They like to experiment, solve puzzles, ask questions. They can be taught through logic games, investigations, and mysteries. *DSL:*
Musical: They can be taught by turning lessons into lyrics, speaking rhythmically, writing rap songs or developing catchy lyrics. *DSL:*
Bodily—Kinesthetic: The student can be taught through physical activity, hands-on learning, acting out, role playing. Tools include equipment and real objects. *DSL:*
Spatial—Visual: They like to draw, do jigsaw puzzles, read maps, or solve complex problems. *DSL*
Interpersonal: The student interacts with others, and DSL includes interviews, journals, newspaper article writing, video conferencing, writing, computer conferencing, e-mail. *DSL*
Intrapersonal: The student can show understanding through books, creative materials, diaries, journals, and reflective logs. *DSL*
Naturalist: Individuals who are high in this type of intelligence are more in tune with nature and are often interested in nurturing, exploring the environment, and learning about other species. *DSL*

THE DELIVERY PHASE

The delivery phase begins with a teacher-directed instruction (large group instruction). During the course of the instructional delivery phase, there are techniques that can be employed that will enhance student achievement. These techniques can be verbal (linguistic) or nonlinguistic. Nonlinguistic representations can include the use of mental imagery. For instance, think to yourself about X, with X representing whatever you wish to visualize. Can you see X in your mind's eye? Ask your students to draw a representation or make a graphic or visual organizer of what they are seeing in their mind.

USING SMALL GROUPS

Small group activity and cooperative learning result in some significant findings because students are thinking, talking, and sharing their ideas so as to promote metacognition. Tips for organizing groups are:

1. Organize groups based on ability level. Students of all ability levels benefit from ability grouping as they have a common baseline conceptual framework of skills
2. Cooperative groups should be kept small so everyone will have a voice. With large groups, some students may be reluctant to speak so they will not contribute to the conversations.
3. Cooperative learning should be applied consistently and systemically with a structure and a purpose.
4. Assign roles and responsibilities to group members. Rotate roles and responsibilities so everyone has an opportunity to take a leadership role for any position.

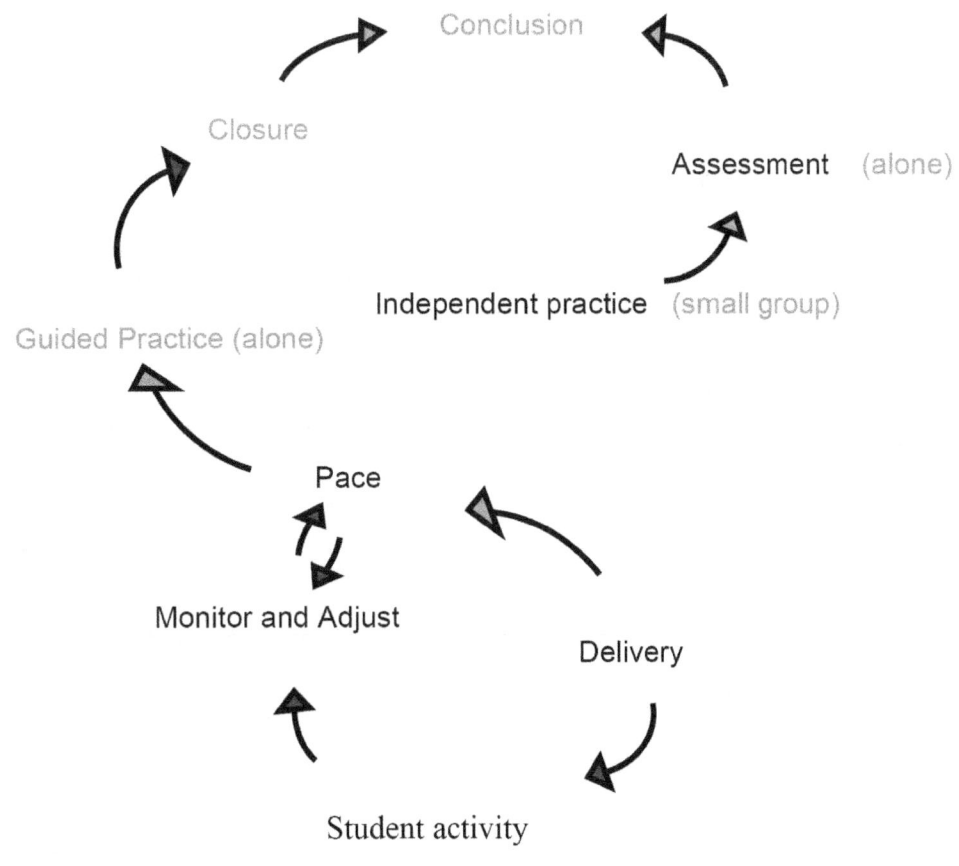

Guided Practice Cycle

After the teacher feels comfortable with the progress of the lesson there may be a point in the lesson for students to start independent practice. The teacher needs to monitor the student's progress and ensure that the student has the knowledge and appropriate skills to do the activity independently and/or at home.

Home learning can involve using massed or distributed practice.

MASSED OR DISTRIBUTED PRACTICE

Massed practice is practicing a new learning, during time periods that are very close together. Sustained practice over time is called distributed practice.

Below is a form that can be used for home learning.

Table 1.8. Home Learning Questions

Questions	Solutions
Brainstorm content-specific terms. Answer the question: The terms are linked by?	
Create a real-world scenario or physical representation to create meaning. Answer the question: How does this apply?	
Compare and contrast related ideas using a graphic organizer or Venn diagram.	
Look up a definition, (e.g., Find the definition for statistics; site your source.)	
Answer the question: Common misconceptions are because?	
Recall previous knowledge by asking: How did I get the answer?	
I know I have it when:	

Reflection

I Know I Have It form

I am learning	
I know one thing about the skill	
Because	
I know I know it by	
I can't show that I know it because I need help with	

REFLECTION

The final task, which concludes the unstructured phase and will be useful for the planning stage, is Consolidation for Closure.

Some strategies are:

1. Ask students to write a three-sentence summary of a lesson.
2. Provide students with a T-Chart and ask them to identify similarities and differences.
3. Have students say what they learned and how it can be applied: How Does It Apply card.
4. Have students show what they learned non-linguistically. The nonlinguistic format will capture key concepts that would be readily obvious to a reader.
5. Evaluate what was learned, and based on what was learned have student use an exit ticket: I hypothesize that:
6. Today I learned . . .
7. I learned X but I still have questions about Y.
8. Provide students with a list of emojis and ask them to circle how they are feeling about the lesson. Provide individual conferences for students who seem sad or confused.
9. Write a tweet about what you learned.
10. Tell a Friend: Write what you learned in a message to a friend.

Consolidation for Closure Dispositions

- Student driven activity
- Students summarize what they perceive is the main ideas, evaluate class processes
- Provides students with opportunities to draw conclusions from the lesson
- Help students understand that Consolidation is a preview for future lessons
- Promote student's problem-solving processing of information

SAMPLE LESSON PLAN

Lesson

Ecosystems: relationships, supports, and interconnectedness

Essential Question

Why does an ecosystem rely on the relationships within it?

Probing Questions

1. How is the ecosystem like other systems that are interrelated?
2. Is your family an ecosystem?
3. If an ecosystem is like a family unit, how do your family members connect with each other? If not, why is it not an ecosystem?
4. How does your family provide support? Is that kind of support the same or different from an ecosystem?

Student Learning Target (Objective)

- I will show the interactions of organisms within an ecosystem by using a Venn diagram and justify my explanation of relationships of organisms in the system.
- I will compare and contrast the essential interdependency of an ecosystem and justify the relationships in the system.
- I will be able to create short stories based on the concepts discussed in this lesson.

Standards to Be Addressed (some standards have been elaborated upon for clarity in this text)

5.1 Scientific Processes: All students will develop problem-solving, decision-making, and inquiry skills, reflected by formulating usable questions and hypotheses, planning experiments, conducting systematic observations, interpreting and analyzing data, drawing conclusions, and communicating results.

Remind Students of Self-Regulation Strategies They Can Use Throughout the Lesson

1. Remind students to use their self-regulated strategies throughout the lesson.
2. Ask two peers before asking the teacher a question.
3. Remind students to make careful observations of their ecosystems. After the observations, they will record their answers in their journals.
4. Encourage students to use research, rubrics, and exemplars to modulate their learning. Rubrics and exemplars will be provided to the students so they can self-regulate and self-modulate their learning.
5. Encourage students to share their learning and work together.
6. Remind students to keep records that describe observations, to carefully distinguish actual observations from ideas and speculations, and write key concepts. They will be instructed to manage their time wisely, as note keeping is a form of self-management and is an important self-regulation strategy.
7. Encourage students to use technology in the classroom (that is, if the district provides laptops or student computer carts).
8. Encourage students to actively seek out information during their independent time.
9. If the students are going to conduct science investigations, they need to keep precise notes about what they are doing, so they can explain the process they used for replication of the experiment. During the process, remind students that you will be questioning them as to why they are doing something. They will need to justify their action.

10. Encourage students to get ideas and help from other people, posters, rubrics, exemplars, or instructional charts in the room. Discuss with them the process of seeking help from others or from collecting information within the room. These two tasks are a form of self-regulation.

Language Arts: 3.2.3 A. Writing as a Process (pre-writing, drafting, revising, editing, post writing)

1. Generate ideas for writing through the process of recalling experiences, active listening to stories, reading, brainstorming, and interactive discussions.
2. Examine real-world examples of writing in various genres, in order to gain an understanding of how authors communicate ideas through form, structure, and "author's voice or literacy style."
3. Use graphic organizers to assist with the development of thoughts. Encourage students to use mind maps or graphic organizers to help conceptualize their ideas.
4. Compose first drafts from pre-writing work. Keep their samples in a performance portfolio, which shows their progress.
5. Revise a rough draft by directing the student to reread the work. Facilitate by encouraging the students to extend meaning, narrow focus, sequence appropriately, expand details, improve openings and closings, and use techniques that create their own literacy style or voice.
6. Participate with peers to comment on and react to each other's writing.
7. Build awareness of ways authors use paragraphs to support meaning.
8. Begin to develop author's voice in their own writing. What is the author saying?
9. Use reference materials such as a dictionary or internet/software resources to revise work.

3.2.3 B. Writing as a Product (resulting in a formal product or publication)

1. Write a descriptive piece, such as a description of a person, place, or object.
2. Present and discuss writing with other students.
3. Apply elements of grade-appropriate rubrics to improve writing.

3.2.3 C. Mechanics, Spelling, Handwriting

1. Use standard English conventions that are developmentally appropriate to the grade level: sentences, punctuation, capitalization, and spelling.
2. Use grade-appropriate knowledge of English grammar and usage to craft writing, such as singular and plural nouns, subject/verb agreement, and appropriate parts of speech.

3.2.3 D. Writing Forms, Audiences, and Purposes (exploring a variety of forms)

1. Write for a variety of purposes (e.g., to inform, entertain, persuade) and audiences (e.g., self, peers, community).
2. Develop fluency by writing daily and for sustained amounts of time.
3. Write the events of a story sequentially.
4. Produce writing that demonstrates the use of a variety of sentence types, such as declarative, interrogative, exclamatory, and imperative.

3.3.3 A. Discussion (small group and whole class)

1. Listen and follow the discussion in order to contribute appropriately.
2. Stay focused on topic.
3. Ensure that all students are participating so they must take turns. Identify roles for the students and have the students rotate their roles throughout the lesson.

4. Support an opinion with details. Support statements with evidence from a text.

3.3.3 C. Word Choice

1. Use vocabulary related to a particular topic.
2. Use words from the word wall.
3. Seek meaning for the vocabulary words

Readiness Set

Teacher states: Have you ever eaten a peanut butter and jelly sandwich? (Another possibility is ham and eggs.) Peanut butter and jelly seem to go well together, don't they? How many students have eaten a ham and egg sandwich? Can you name sandwiches that you can make yourself that go well together? (Students may name ham and cheese, bologna and cheese, cream cheese and jelly, grilled cheese and bacon, etc.)

Teacher should accept any answer the student shares, as long as they answer "two items that go together." Teacher states: What if you can't make the sandwich by yourself, what would you do? When was the last time you received help from someone (or you may say an unexpected source, depending upon the age level of the student)?

Teacher states: Today we are going to talk about two points: First, we will discuss how things are related or how things go together in the environment. Secondly, we will discuss how we receive help and our reaction to that helpfulness.

Teacher states: Let's think about those two questions (teacher repeats the two questions as reinforcement to non-auditory learners). (Teacher note: After you reflect upon the two questions and a very brief discussion is held between the teacher and the students, direct the students to place a one-sentence entry in their journal, noting their own thoughts about the two questions). Teacher states: You will have four minutes to enter a sentence or two about your feelings regarding these two questions. After four minutes, we will share what each of you wrote with your classmates.

As students share their sentence entries, their classmates may reflect upon the entries in a round-circle discussion forum or the teacher may choose to break the class into groups and have each student read their entry to a group of five or six peers. (Teacher note: Rules of active listening should be posted prior to the beginning of the readings and a posting of skills for note taking.) It is important for the teacher to observe the writings, as the students should begin to form "relationships" from their notes and from the discussions.

Consolidation for Closure (exit ticket examples)

This technique shows the teacher what students are thinking and what they have learned at the end of a lesson. It is used after a lesson is taught. Students are given a "ticket" and asked to fill it out by answering a question, solving a problem, or a responding to what they've learned.

Exit Ticket	TODAY I LEARNED:
Exit Ticket	TODAY I LEARNED:

Use exit tickets at the end of class to:

- Check students' understanding by having them summarize key points from the lesson
- Verify that students can solve a problem or answer a significant question based on the lesson
- Emphasize the essential question for the day's lesson
- Have students ask questions they still have about the lesson
- See if students can apply the content in a new way
- Formulate guided groups for students who did not demonstrate understanding after the lesson
- Create extensions for students who demonstrate mastery after the lesson

REFERENCES

Angelo, T. A., and Cross, K. P. (1993). *Classroom Assessment Techniques: A Handbook for College Teachers* (2nd ed.). San Francisco: Jossey-Bass.

Bloom, B. S. (1956). *Taxonomy of Educational Objectives: The Classification of Educational Goals*

Handbook I: Cognitive Domain. New York: David McKay Company.

Bookheimer, S. Y., Zeffiro, T.A., Blaxton, T. A., Giaillard, P. W. and Theodore. W. H . (2000). Activation of language cortex with automatic speech tasks. *Neurology, 55* (8).

Bush, G. (1990). Presidential Proclamation 6158. (Library of Congress), available at: http://leweb.loc.gov/loc/brain/proclaim.html

Cowley, G., and Underwood, A. (1998). Memory. *Newsweek, 131* (May).

Dewey, John. (1895). The Theory of Emotion (1) Emotional Attitudes. *Psychological Review* 1.

Dewey, John. (1896). The reflex arc concept in psychology. *Psychological Review* (3).

Dewey, John. (1902). *The Child and The Curriculum and The School and Society*. Chicago: The University of Chicago Press.

Dewey, John. (1910). *How We Think*. Lexington, MA: D.C. Heath.

Dewey, John (1915). *Schools of Tomorrow*. New York: Dutton Press.

Dewey, John. (1916). The Relationship of Thought and Its Subject Matter, Chapter 2 in *Essays in Experimental Logic*. Chicago, University of Chicago.

Dewey, John. (1933). How We Think, A Restatement of The Relation of Reflective Thinking. *The Educative Process*. Boston: D. C. Heath.

Dewey, John. (1938). *Experience and Education*. New York: Collier Books.

Diamond, M., and Hopson, J. (1998). *Magic Trees of the Mind: How to Nurture Your Child's Intelligence, Creativity and Healthy Emotions from Birth through Adolescence*. New York: Penguin Putnam.

Ebbinghaus, H. (1885). *Memory: A Contribution to Experimental Psychology*, Henry A. Ruger and Clare E. Bussenius, Trans. (1913). Originally published in New York by Teachers College in the History of Psychology, as internet resource developed by Christopher D. Green, New Your University, Toronto, Ontario.

Gazzaniga, M.S., and LeDoux, J.E. (1978). *The Integrated Mind*. New York: Plenum

Hermann, D. J., Weingartnerm H., Searleman, A., and McEvoy, C. (1992). *Memory Improvement: Implications for Memory*. New York: Springer-Verlag.

Holloway, John (2000, November) How does the brain learn science? *Educational Leadership* 58 3.

Hunter, M. (1979, October). Teaching is decision making. *Educational Leadership*.

Hunter, M. (1982). *Mastery Teaching*. El Segundo, CA: TIP Publications.

Huttenlocher, P. R., and Dabholkan, A. S. (1997). Regional differences in synaptogenesis in human cerebral cortex. *The Journal of Comparative Neurology, 387*.

Jensen, Eric (1998). How Julie's Brain Learns. *Educational Leadership. 51* (3)

Jensen, E. (2010). *Different Brains, Different Learners: How to Reach the Hard to Reach*. Thousand Oaks, CA: Corwin Press.

Krug, Mark. (1972) *What Will Be Taught—The Nextade*. Itasca, IL: F. E. Peacock, Publishers, Inc.

LeDoux, J.E. (1994). Emotion, memory and the brain. *Scientific American 270*, 50–57.

LeDoux, JE (1996) *The Emotional Brain*. New York: Simon & Schuster.

LeDoux, J.E. (2000) *Synaptic Self: How the Brain Becomes Who We Are*. New York; Viking

LeDoux, J.E. (2000). Emotion circuits in the brain. *Annual Review Neuroscience 23*, 155–184.

Lepore, F. (2001). Dissecting Genius: Einstein's Brain and the Search for the Neural Basis of Intellect, The Dana Foundation, January 1.

Marzano, R., Pickering, W., and Pollock, J. (2001). *Classroom Instruction That Works*. Alexandria, VA: Association for Supervision and Curriculum Development.

Marzano, R. J. (2007). *The Art and Science of Teaching: A Comprehensive Framework for Effective Instruction*. Alexandria, VA: Association for Supervision and Curriculum Development.

Mireles, Selina Vásquez, Westbrook, Theresa, Ward, Debra D., Goodson, Joshua, and Jung, Jae Hak. (2013, Spring). Implementing Pre-Homework in the Developmental Mathematics Classroom. Research & Teaching in Developmental, *29*(3).

Mueller, C. M., and Dweck, C. S. (1998). Intelligence praise can undermine motivation and performance. *Journal of Personality and Social Psychology*, 75(1), 33–52.

Praxis. (1995). Paper presented at the Annual Meeting of the American Education Research Association, San Francisco, CA, April 18–22, 1995.

Ramey, C.T., and Ramey, S.L. (1996, February). At risk does not mean doomed. *National Health/Education Consortium Occasional Paper, #4*. Paper presented at the meeting of the American Association of Science.

Sousa, David. (2000). *How the Brain Learns*. Thousand Oaks, CA: Corwin Press.

Sousa, David. (2001). *How the Special Needs Brain Learns*. Thousand Oaks, CA: Corwin Press.

Stiggins, R. (2005). From formative assessment to assessment FOR learning: A path to success in standards-based schools. *Phi Delta Kappan, 86*, 324–328.

Stiggins, R. (2005). *Student-Involved Assessment FOR Learning*. Upper Saddle River, NJ: Pearson Education.

Stiggins, R., and Chappuis, J. (2005). Using student-involved classroom assessment to close achievement gaps. *Theory into Practice, 44*, 11–18.

Tomlinson, C., and McTighe, J. (2006). *Integrating Differentiation and Understanding by Design: Connecting Content and Kids*. Alexandria, VA: Association for Supervision and Curriculum Development.

Willingham, D. T. (2010). *Why Don't Students Like School? A Cognitive Scientist Answers Questions About How the Mind Works and What It Means for the Classroom*. San Francisco: Jossey-Bass.

Wolfe, Pat. (1999). Revisiting effective teaching. *Educational Leadership 56* (3) 61–61.

Wolfe, Patricia (2001). *Brain Matters; Translating Research Into Classroom Practice*. Alexandria, VA: ASCD.

Willis, J. (2006). *Research-Based Strategies to Ignite Student Learning: Insights from a Neurologist and Classroom Teacher*. Alexandria, VA: Association for Supervision and Curriculum Development.

2

Middle Stage of Learner's Brain Model
Assessments

FOCUS OF THE CHAPTER

This chapter will focus on how to use assessments, ways to develop assessments and assessment activities, which will ensure that lessons successfully monitor student progress. By using formative and summative assessments and data to drive instruction, assessments data is provided for lesson planning. The focus of the chapter is on analyzing data so the teacher is not "data rich" and "analysis poor."

INTRODUCTION

Too often there is a dichotomy that testing is the teacher's friend or foe. It is the teacher's foe if a teacher is evaluated on a standards-based assessment although her students are reading two to three years below grade level and expected to meet or exceed proficiency.

Assessments and testing can be the teacher's friend if the assessments are used for lesson planning and data collection. This chapter will discuss and provide activities on how assessments can determine what was effectively taught. Additionally, assessments protocols that can be used for promoting long-term retention will be discussed.

PROBING QUESTIONS

1. How will the information from the assessments be used?
2. How will my assessments be tied to standards?
3. How will I know if my assessments provide data to me about my students and if they are learning throughout the lesson?
4. What are assessment activities I can use that incorporate different learning modalities?

GUIDING PRINCIPLES

Tests and assessments can be a teacher's friend or foe. They can be the teacher's foe if a student takes a test, does poorly, and becomes discouraged, frustrated, or upset.

Table 2.1. Activity Sheet

How will the information from the assessments be used? (In essence, why am I doing this assessment?)
What standards are addressed by this assessment?
How will I know if my assessments provide data to me about my students and if they are learning throughout the lesson?
What are assessment activities I can use that incorporate different learning modalities?

However, tests and assessments can be our friend if the teacher uses information, for example, checking for understanding or formative assessments from the test for monitoring and adjusting the learning. The assessment strategies are done throughout the instructional period to assess if the student knows or understands the material, thereby enabling the teacher to pace his or her lesson.

Additionally, tests can be used for improvement of learning or as a way for students to study. In the former case, assessments are done during the instructional period by the teacher, and in the latter, strategies are done during the time set aside for homework by the student as a strategy to help improve his or her learning. Finally, if the goal is to develop self-regulated learners, it is the student who must engage in assessment to promote the process of regulation.

The question becomes: How can teachers employ various strategies to help promote student learning by using assessments or tests?

STUDENT USE OF ASSESSMENTS

Often the conventional thinking of assessments is that teachers provide information, and an assessment is given so the teacher can determine if the instruction was effective. This protocol directs the process from teacher to student. How can the teacher help the student to direct or assess his or her own learning and promote the use of tests and assessments for the process of student self-regulation? If the student were to engage in such a protocol, one would develop a feedback loop emanating from the teacher to the student back to the teacher. The critical fact of this kind of a feedback loop is that the student uses assessments for the purpose of self-regulated learning.

The first step in the process would be to ensure that students understand and employ self-regulated learning strategies. In order for this to occur, the teachers must teach self-regulating learning strategies. Teachers can model the process whenever

Table 2.2. Activity: Assessment for Learning or of Learning

Assessment for learning	Assessment of learning
My assessments measure learning by	My assessments will be used for learning by
I will use the data for lesson planning by	I will use the data for student learning by

possible and explain to students what she is doing so the student will understand that self-regulated learning requires using various strategies.

As discussed earlier, the self-regulated classroom provides rubrics, exemplars, meaningful feedback, journals, work folders, portfolios to environmentally construct the learning environment. However, just the construction of the environment by posting information will not be enough as a student may soon ignore the information as it will blend into the classroom and not be seen as a meaningful resource.

The teacher must therefore tell the student that it is his/her responsibility to promote their own learning through self-regulation and use the resources in the classroom. If the teacher relies on summative assessments to determine student progress, it may be too late. Therefore the teacher must encourage students to take responsibility for their own learning as they are learning.

The teacher may tell the class: I want to remind you that throughout the lesson I will be monitoring our progress but I also want you to monitor your own progress.

I will provide instruction throughout the lesson and talk about what strategies I am using, but I also ask that you monitor your progress in one of two ways

1. Throughout the period, refer to the rubrics that you have been provided or the rubrics and exemplars that are posted throughout the room to assess your progress.
2. While doing your home learning, continue to use the rubrics and exemplars to assess your learning as well as the use of assessments. The assessments can be short quizzes.

The promoting of self-regulation concept for students is necessary even though some students are more inclined to self-regulate their learning than others.

As a teacher teaches the lesson, students should be reminded that if they are having difficulties, they are to seek out help in other ways before they come to the teacher. This notion of "two" or "three before me" promotes students seeking resolutions to their problems before going to the teacher first. The "two before me" can involve students talking to other students, using the Internet to research their answer, or using reference charts, etc., in the classroom as examples of strategies. In this fashion they are seeking alternative ways to resolve the problem before they go to the teacher.

For students in the lower grades, a rubric, which can include pictures, can be developed for them to use in the assessment of their own learning. Below is an example of a Reflection Sheet for self-regulation and a rubric developed by Christine Castle, teacher in Elizabeth Public Schools. She uses this with her first-grade students and they love the visuals. Since the Jersey Shore is a big part of life in New Jersey, it is no surprise the students would love a rubric that includes fish.

REFLECTION

What Self-Regulation Strategies Do I Want the Students to Know?

What Strategies Will I Show for Student Self-Regulation?

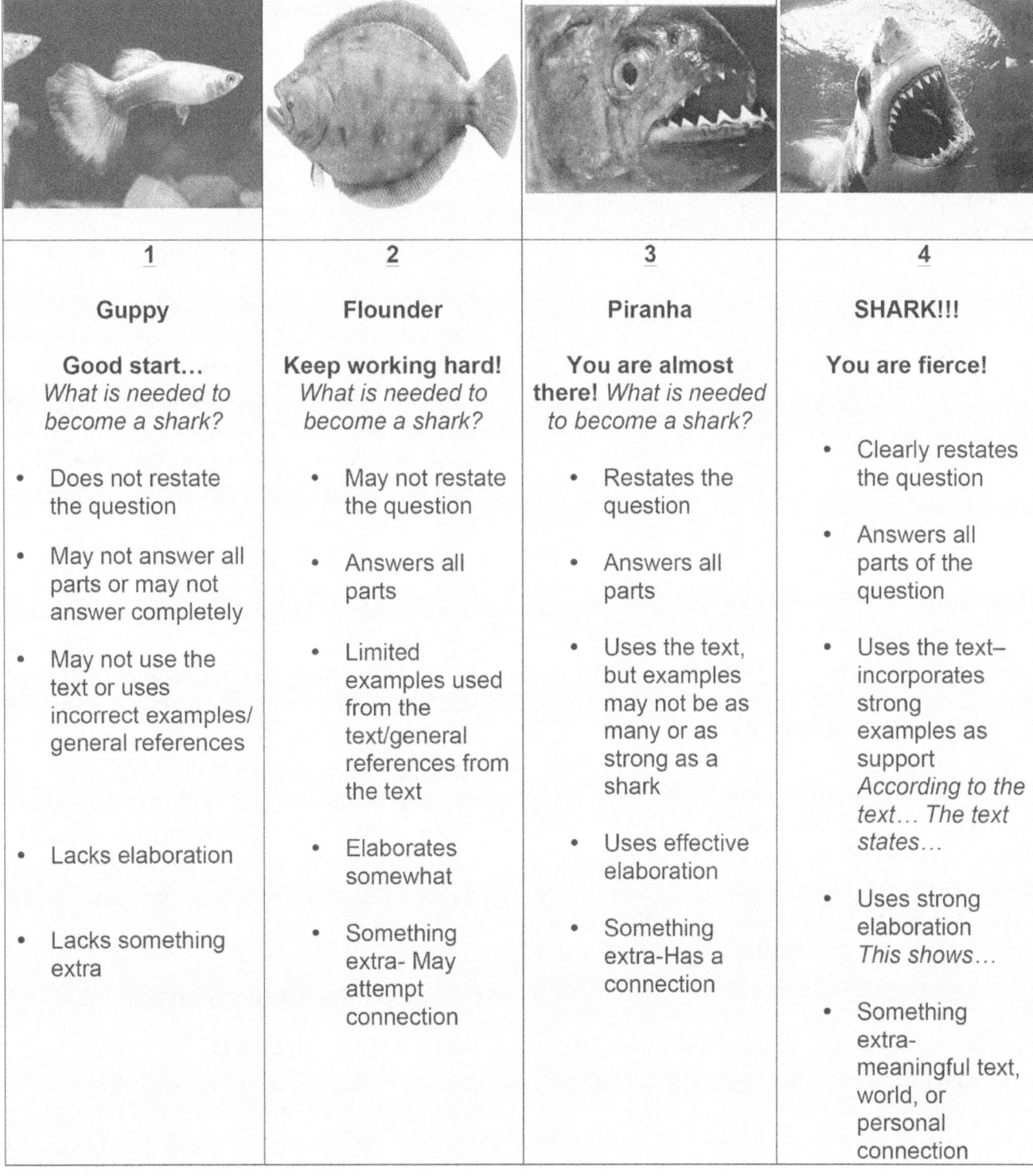

Open-Ended Responses

USING ASSESSMENTS AND TESTS FOR LEARNING

The question: How can the teacher make the lesson more successful? The answer: Monitor student progress using formative and summative assessments. Below is a sample lesson plan that incorporates assessments to drive instruction.

Teacher's Name: Chris Barbiere

Lesson: Healthy Living (Wellness)

Unit Topic: Circulatory System

Grade Level: 8

BACKGROUND: CROSS-CURRICULAR WITH HEALTH UNIT ON FITNESS TRAINING AND A HEALTHY HEART

HEALTHY HEART (OVERVIEW)

This health unit deals with wellness and maintaining a healthy heart using three forms of exercise, Aerobic, Anaerobic, and Flexibility and a healthy diet to maintain a healthy heart.

The students will perform each type of exercise while taking heart rate readings, creating statistical representations of the data and comparing each type of exercise to understand the relationship of exercise and health and wellness. They will gather research on exercise as it relates to the promotion of a healthy heart.

The students will analyze their diet to expose the components of their diet that may lead to high cholesterol levels, obesity, and a reduction in heart health. They will gather research on heart health diets.

Students will create a Venn diagram showing how exercise and diet contribute to wellness and a healthy heart using their research notes.

Essential Questions

What is wellness and how does it relate to healthful living?
What role does exercise and diet play in healthful living?
How is exercise and diet related to wellness?

Student Learning Target (Objectives)

- I will be able to explain five of the major factors associated with cardiovascular disease and justify my answers with research.
- I will be able to explain and justify the role of exercise and diet as it relates to wellness.
- I will be able to create a diet plan and exercise plan for me based on my research and findings.

Demonstration of Student Learning (DSL)

- I will be able to create a healthy exercise and diet plan.
- Given a healthy teenager and senior citizen, I will be able to analyze their data, compare and contrast their vascular wellness, and explain how they are the same and different.
- Given a cardiovascular disease, I will be able to construct a T-Chart listing symptoms of the disease and justifying my response. I will be able to create a plan of exercise and diet to resolve the cardiovascular disease.

Standards to Be Addressed (CCSS)

HEALTH

Standard 2.1 seeks to address these concerns by supporting the concept of health promotion and disease prevention. The underlying principle of this standard is that all students need to learn to take enhancing behaviors that support lifelong wellness.

Indicator 2.1-11: Analyze a health profile to determine strengths and potential health risks resulting from risk factors and health-enhancing behaviors.

Indicator 2.1-11: Analyze a health profile to determine strengths and potential health risks resulting from risk factors and health-enhancing

CONTENT AREA: Health [AU: ?]

GRADE: 8

UNIT#: 1

UNIT NAME: Wellness

Student Learning Objective (New Jersey) Number: 3, 8, 9, 12

Table 2.3. To Promote Student Self-Regulation
Rubric for assessing student work (Explain to the students that the rubric is used for their self regulation)
(Have students peer edit using the rubric)

Developing	Need Improvement	Targeted	Exceeds Targeted
Student can list facts or a wellness plan. Student can list facts related to the value of exercise. No connection between wellness and exercise.	Student is unable to analyze the facts about wellness and exercise to show their relationship.	Student analyzes research to justify a relationship between exercise, wellness, and an effective cardiovascular system.	Uses research to create a plan for a healthy heart combining exercise and diet.

WELLNESS

1. Research on wellness and exercise is provided and students are encouraged to use it to supplement their own research.
2. Exercise plans of athletes are provided as examples.
3. Wellness plans are provided as exemplars.
4. Information about "healthy heart" is provided and students are requested to use it.
5. Grading rubrics provided to students to use for self-regulation

Readiness Set (10 minutes)

This activity begins the Readiness Stage (please see below) of the Learner's Brain Model.

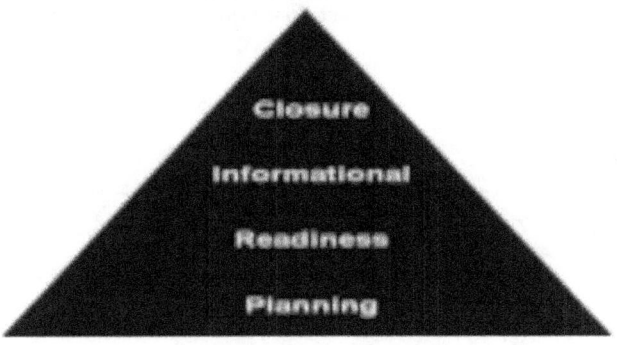

Learner's Brain Model

Students write their answers to questions.

1. What do you know about Heart Attacks? (*This question promotes developing student readiness and background knowledge as well as activating their prior knowledge. As students share out, it will provide additional information for students and give the teacher valuable information.*)
2. Have you seen ads on television about exercise and a healthy heart or on diet and a healthy heart? Write what the ad was about or what information the ad tried to convey.
3. Do you know anyone who had a heart attack or stroke? If you do, what happened? (*This question stimulates prior knowledge and helps to promote meaning and make sense.*) Have they made changes in their diet or exercise since the heart attack?
4. Tell your neighbor if exercise can be good for you? (*This question will help students see the relationship between health, wellness, exercise, and nutrition to promote cross-curricular studies.*)
5. Ask athletes to write about their exercise and diet plans. After their plans are discussed, the teacher will ask the class: What do you notice about their exercise and diet plans?

6. Why do some folks have "special" diets?
7. How much exercise is needed for a "healthy" heart?
8. Can only exercise prevent heart attacks?
9. Can only a healthy diet prevent heart attacks?

Students then engage in a pair-share activity to discuss their ideas followed by quick class discussion. During the class discussion, the teacher discusses the relationship between exercise, diet and healthy heart.

Teacher observation from the group discussions (please list several observations):

The purpose of the questions is to stimulate prior knowledge in one of two ways: one, by students focusing on exercise and health; two, to show the relationship between diet and exercise either by personal experience or via secondhand information.

Additionally, the cross-curricular questions are tied to the realization of heart attacks and how to prevent them. Since exercise is one way to prevent heart disease, students will have prior knowledge about healthful living and the value of exercise. More importantly, they will begin to see the relationship between diet and exercise as being effective and not just diet or exercise.

Other Cross-Curricular Questions:

Alternate Readiness Set

Students in the elementary grades can do a tracing of their body outline and attach it to a wall in the classroom. Ask a volunteer to place a picture or drawing of a heart in the correct location on the outline. *(Foreshadowing of what is to come—a lesson about the heart; assessing prior knowledge.)*

Ask each student to place a hand over his/her heart to see if they can feel it beating. Ask the students to jump up and down and then place their hand over their heart to see if they feel any difference. Ask the class: What happened to your heart after you exercised?

Use a stethoscope to allow each child to hear his/her own heartbeat and that of another classmate. Explain that the sound means that the heart (a pump) is pumping blood throughout the body. Explain that the heart is a muscle. Ask students what they do to keep their muscles in shape. What can they do to keep their heart in shape?

Ask the students if they exercised today. Make the connection that exercise for the body is exercise for the heart and explain how exercise helps the heart to pump more effectively. Brainstorm other ways to keep the heart healthy and list them on the board. The teacher will finish the activity by having each student write "I will keep my heart healthy by. . . ."

Activity variation:

Create a healthy diet. Ask students if they eat any of these foods? If not, what foods do they eat? Do they eat healthy snacks?

Other possible activities or activities using Multiple Pathways

Table 2.4. Fieldbook Activity

Student Learning Target:

Demonstration of Student Learning

Readiness Set example
I believe this is effective because:

Readiness Set example
I believe this is effective because:

After the Readiness Set

Next, the Student Learning Target (objective) and Demonstration of Student Learning (DSL) is introduced to the class. The teacher engaged the students' prior knowledge by saying, "We all have seen or know someone affected by a heart attack, so today we learn about wellness and the major factors associated with cardiovascular disease and the consequences related to it. To ensure that I know you understand the concepts being taught, you will be asked to compare and contrast two age groups and justify how they can prevent heart attacks." *(This task promotes forethought, the first step in self-regulation. Keep this in mind because throughout the lesson you will be provided information to use for your Venn diagram.)*

The teacher reminds the class that we have two objectives for today's lesson:

- I will be able to identify, analyze, and justify major factors associated with wellness.
- I will be able to create a wellness plan incorporating exercise and diet.

Demonstration of Student Learning (DSL)

I will be able to compare and contrast exercise and diet plans between teenagers and adults to determine the elements of an effective plan.

"Prior to beginning today's lesson, I will share with you an action plan and the rubric which we used to assess your assignment. We will be working in small groups and I will be circulating around the room to provide guidance and support."

The teacher will convey this information to the students so they know teacher expectations and that the teacher will be providing support throughout the lesson. The importance of self-regulation strategies is suggested.

INSTRUCTIONAL INPUT (THIS BEGINS THE INFORMATIONAL STAGE OF THE LEARNER'S BRAIN MODEL)

Modeling

Students are being required to create an action plan that if followed closely may help to promote wellness and prevent cardiovascular disease.

An example of an Action Plan is shown as an example so that students can self-regulate and the rubric that will be used for grading is modeled. Resources will be provided in the room so students can self-regulate their learning.

Students will present their Action Plan so they can be creative in their approach and use any appropriate format—written account, song, poem / short story, blog, wiki space, play, SMART board file, PowerPoint, video, radio interview etc. The critical factor is that the students will be taught to use self-regulated learning strategies throughout the lesson.

Large Group Activity

The teacher will provide information to the students about wellness, diet, heart disease, and the value of exercise. After the large group instruction activity, small groups of three to four students will be determined based on interest, teacher selection, or student selection. Students will be asked to use the resources in the room to self-regulate.

Small Group Activity

Students will work in small groups for approximately 20 minutes to read and discuss three articles. They will use a jigsaw approach in that each student will have one article to read after which they will share information from the article with the remaining students in their group.

Activities (20 minutes)

Students will work in groups to discuss three articles.

1. American Heart Association article on Healthy Heart
2. Peer-reviewed magazine article on Diet and Exercise as it relates to wellness
3. Two articles from national newspaper, for example, *New York Times*, *Washington Post*, or *Guardian* (UK) on Childhood Obesity and Cardiovascular Disease
4. Students research wellness, exercise, and diet in which they will be the "expert" and share their finding with the class

Articles are assigned/differentiated for individual reading according to student's reading level. Students are reminded to keep in mind the essential question while reading.

Early finishers use the Internet to get additional research for their assignment.

During the small group activity, teacher will monitor groups. Teacher will ask probing questions as well as reflective questions to ensure that the students are staying focused on the task at hand as well as obtaining information necessary for them to do their report.

The teacher may say: "As you pair-share your ideas about wellness, diet, heart disease, exercise, and healthy heart, who can share with me what was discussed?" During the discussion, the teacher will refer back to the objective to keep the students focused. "Don't forget today we are learning about wellness, the heart, heart disease, diet, and exercise."

Or the teacher can remind the students that: Today you are learning about wellness and the impact of heart disease and exercise and you will be held responsible for comparing and contrasting information. You will need to obtain details and facts to be able to justify your answers. As you work on your assignment, remember to ask yourself "why" questions so you are able to take the information and think how you will be able to create your own action plan.

Teachers who use strategies that focus students on higher-order thinking skills, give consistent, timely, and process-oriented feedback, and work to extend students' language skills, tend to have students who achieve more academically. (See the following research: Hamre and Pianta, 2005; Justice, Meier, and Walpole, 2005; Meehan, Hughes, and Cavell, 2003; Taylor, Pearson, Peterson, and Rodriguez, 2003, in Allen et al., 2013.)

Check for Understanding

Teacher circulates throughout class and uses informal questioning and graphic organizer completion to check for individual understanding. As students are reading the articles, the teacher will ask: What is the most important concept in the article and why is it important?

Or the teacher can use a Five-Sentence Summary where students summarize what they learned in three sentences. The teacher will review the Five-Sentence Summary to determine if the students are extracting the critical elements of the paper.

Assessments

Formative Assessment: completion of closure activity and exit cards on the major theme of the day. Formative assessment will involve:

Guided Practice and Monitoring of Small Groups (15)

Students read the article and use the graphic organizer provided to summarize the important points. Students can also use the Cornell Notes system for note taking while reading the article.

Students meet in groups to discuss their articles and complete a chart by listing the similar information contained in all of the articles and three points that they did not have. Students are guided to include important points that may help answer the essential question.

Students are asked to discuss in their groups:

1. How did the articles help with your understanding of wellness, the role of diet and exercise? Why?
2. What do you not agree with from the articles? Make a Venn diagram of exercise, diet in relation to wellness.
3. Why is wellness dependent on multiple factors?

Teacher circulates to each group and asks questions to aid in comprehension, guide discussion, and check for understanding using singling, sampling, or choral responses.

Small group discussions are conducted with the teacher on the major points, including how the gathered information may help students create their action plan. Signaling and sampling to check for understanding will enable the teacher to determine if the students have the main concepts or if instruction is needed.

Examples of checks of understanding can include:

Strategy	Example
1. Hand Signals: Thumbs Up/Down; 2. Three, two, one finger	The teacher asks students to display a hand signal to indicate their understanding. • I understand and can explain it (e.g., *thumbs up, 3 fingers*). • I do not yet understand (e.g., *thumbs down, 1 finger*). • I'm not completely sure (e.g., *thumb sideways, 2 fingers*).
3. Whiteboard	The teacher asks the students a question during the lesson. • Students have time to process the question and write responses on the whiteboard. • Students hold up the whiteboards and display their answers. • The teacher checks the whiteboards for student answers. If many have the correct answer, the teacher can have students with the correct answer talk to students who did not have the correct answer. If everyone has a correct answer, the teacher can read the answer and ask everyone if they agree. Since students may not be able to see all the whiteboards, they will hear the choral response and determine that their answer is the correct answer. • The teacher restates the correct answer with the whole class. • Since not everyone can see all the whiteboards, the teacher should be mindful of sharing information with the whole class, so they hear the correct answers and so they know that they are "on track."
4. Sixty-second paper	Students summarize the main ideas they got from their classmates' discussions during the small group activity or after the teacher reviews their choral responses. The students can review their one-minute summary with their classmates. (*It would be an effective strategy for students to engage in dialogue and metacognition.*)
5. Cloudy point / sunny point	*Cloudy point:* Students write about the point they had the most difficulty understanding during the lesson. Or students tell their partner what they had difficulty with during the lesson. *Sunny Point:* Students can write or say what they enjoyed most about the information they gathered during the small group activity or from the large group lesson. This information can lead to discussions, justifications of responses, debates, pros/cons, or other kinds of activities.
6. I have a question; who has the answer?	Students who have a muddy point can raise a question for someone to answer and ask: Who has the answer? Classmates can provide answers to the questions that are posed.
7. Sampling	Sampling means posing questions to the total group, allowing students time to think, and then calling on class members representative of the ability strata of the group (most able, average, least able). Be mindful that the person selected is only one person so ensure that the person is a representative sample.
8. Letter	Explain in one paragraph what you learned today.
9. Pro/Con	Students who support (pro) stand up; students who disagree (con) remain seated. Students who agree explain to the students who disagree to try and convince them to change their mind.

As the teacher does the checks for understanding, and depending on the information that is gained, the lesson can be adjusted accordingly. The whole purpose of the checking for understanding is to monitor student learning to adjust the instruction based on monitoring.

The natural flow from information gathering to lesson planning would be the evolution of student engagement activities or differentiation of instruction based on the feedback that is received.

After the instructional delivery stage, teacher will do a closing activity. There are many closing activities that can be done.

Agree/disagree pair share	Teacher can have students who agree with a point of view discuss it with students who disagree with the point which is made. The teacher can also engage the students by having them develop pros (agree) and cons (disagree) to the comments made. A home learning activity would be to justify all the "agree" statements with research.
Agree/disagree debate teams	Based on the agree/disagree information, teachers can make two debate teams—one team of agree and one team of disagree. Each team will develop questions based on their point of view to ask the other team. Students need to have research to justify their answers.
Student-generated test questions	Have students devise possible test questions as a home learning assignment. Review what was submitted and provide feedback to the students so that they have a better understand of the assessment process and where they can improve. What students suggest as questions is an indication of what they think is important. Use the information from the students to plan future lessons.
Student-generated test questions with rubric	Consider letting students apply criteria (even creating a test's scoring rubric) for essay questions that they develop. The development of rubrics will help students understand the criteria for assessment at several levels.
Find a place	The teacher establishes four areas for students to use for the activity. The areas are strongly agree, agree, strongly disagree, or disagree. Students go to one of the four areas to vote on how they feel. They can have a discussion with their colleagues while at the area to assess if their opinion still remains the same. While they are in their four areas, students can list all of the reasons for their voting. The next step would be to have them come up with a list of phrases captured in their discussions.
My study list	Each team can make a list of words or concepts to review or study that can be used for a home learning assignment. Students will be required to develop a definition and justification for each word or phrase.
Key words	Students give the teacher a list of key words and concepts from the lesson. A follow-up activity is to make the key words part of "My Study List."
30-second summary	Students write a short summary of what they learned and give it to the teacher on their way out of the class; it then becomes their "exit ticket. The teacher can also make it a 60-second or 90- second summary
Five-sentence summary	Students capture the essence of the lesson by writing what they learned in five sentences.
LCA	A three-sentence summary with: one sentence is what I learned today (L), one sentence is what I am confused about (C), and one sentence is how I will apply the information (A)
My learning concept map	Concept map. Based on the lesson, students diagram the relationships of the concepts that were taught.
For/against	Students make a "T" chart and write down the pros (for) and cons (against) of the concepts taught.
"Ticket to Leave"	Exit ticket or ticket to leave. Students summarize what they learned on 3 x 5 index card.
What I know and What I wonder	Students write what they know (learned) on the front of an index card and what they wonder or need extra help with on the back to the card.
Today I learned	Students write a short summary of what they learned.
Interview questions	Students write a list of interview questions (facts they want to know).
Baseball	The students will earn a single, double, triple, or home run by: Single: Write one thing you learned today. Double: Write two things you learned today. Triple: Write three things you learned today. Home run: Write four things you learned today.

Multiple Pathways (Intelligences)

Linguistic

- Students will develop an inventive dialogue between a teenager and a senior citizen about healthy habits. They will have research to support their claims.
- Have the student read an article on wellness, healthy heart, diet, and exercise as it relates to wellness, then have the students lead a class discussion.
- Student will use information from multiple websites to support a point of view and write a blog about their findings.
- Students choose their Action Plan Product and write an essay on health in their journal, which will be reviewed by the teacher the next day.

Logical–Mathematical

- Students will use a peer-reviewed journal article on wellness or cardiovascular disease statistics and graph the information. They write an interpretive statement about the graph.
- Based on information they learned in class, students will develop a graph to show the relationship of exercise, wellness, and a healthy heart.
- Students will create a puzzle based on the mathematical concepts they learned.

Musical

- Students will create a rap song about "Wellness," "The Healthy Heart."
- Students choose their Action Plan Product and create a video about wellness.
- Students will use Garage Band to create a song about exercise and nutrition.

Bodily–Kinesthetic

- Students create an interpretive dance about nutrition and healthy hearts.
- Create an activity about a healthy heart and write a script that is supported by research about wellness.
- Students create a "healthy heart" maze with "stop" points that have information about heart health.

Spatial–Visual

- Students will create a graphic organizer about exercise and nutrition for a healthy heart. Research will be provided to support the various points in the graphic organizer.
- Students choose their Action Plan Product and construct a graphic model based on their plan.

Interpersonal

- Create a script for an interview. Students will work with partners to conduct their interview. In order to prepare for the interview they must have a fact sheet.
- Students will create a FAQ list based on information from interviewing fellow students.
- Students will work in pairs to create a "newspaper" article on what they learned.
- Students will develop a board game for the class.

Intrapersonal

- Students will write a paragraph on what the lesson meant to them.
- Student will make an entry into their daily reflective journal about the lesson and create a personal plan for health.

Naturalist

- Students will compare and contrast two articles related to the environment.
- Students will write about the impact of the environment on health.

Table 2.7. Additional Closure Activities

Tell Doc (or substitute your name, i.e., Ms. X)	Have students write on an index card what they learned today and give the card to you on the way out of class.
Tell your absent friend what they missed today	Have students write three things they learned today to share with an absent classmate.
Tell Mom/Dad/Grandma/ Grandpa what they missed today	Select anyone from the list to have the student write to about what they learned today and why it is important.
Draw a picture	Have students draw a picture or graphic organizer of what they learned in class.
Tell SAM	Have students write on an index card why today's lessons made Sense And had Meaning (SAM)
I want to tell you a secret	My secret is that today I learned . . .
Send a text	Send a text to your friend about what you learned today.
Game plan	Write what you learned today as a game plan for tomorrow's lesson. For example: I learned this because I can use it tomorrow when I am learning X.

Accommodations

1. Teacher will provide differentiated reading assignments based on student reading levels.
2. Recorded passage for student X will be made available to the student.
3. Teacher will provide different levels of graphic organizers for students with Individualized Educational Plans.
4. Teacher will use small group instruction time for individualized attention.

Assessments

Formative Assessment: completion of closure activity and exit cards on the major theme of the day. Please see examples above.

Consolidation for Closure (10 minutes)

Students reflect on

1. How did today's lesson help with my Action Plan?
2. What do I need to do tomorrow?
3. The Essential Question: What can I add to the answer?
4. Where am I on the assignment rubric?

Student will use an exit ticket to answer one of the four questions above (overt closure).

Student will discuss with their partner/group (covert closure).

Independent Practice

Students continue with the formulation of their Wellness Plan at home and must have one component of the plan completed by tomorrow. Students will come to class tomorrow with an "Admit Ticket" which will list any questions, concerns, barriers they had while doing their home learning. The admit slips will be collected by the teacher, read aloud, and be used to begin discussion for the lesson.

After all of the above has been done, there are two distinct approaches to using assessments to promote learning. One approach is to use assessments for learning at the end (summative) and the other is to use assessments for learning during the class (formative).

Assessments

If teachers decide to use multiple-choice types of assessments then there is a checklist below that teachers can use to determine the kinds of questions that are being asked.

In the first column the teacher keeps a tally of the kinds of questions that were being asked. What will the students be doing?

In the second column is Revised Bloom's Taxonomy, which provides guidance to the teacher on the kind of question that is being asked.

The action column is the student's cognition level, which is being asked to perform.

The last column provides sample questions. What is the level of cognition I am seeking?

At the conclusion of the activity, the teacher can assess how many types of questions were used at each level? What does that tell you?

The chart can also be used to rework the question posed to a different level. To guide the teacher, there are sample questions to ask and actions that can be done.

The goal is to help the teacher see the kinds of questions being asked and how the questions can be "upgraded" to a different level by changing the question being asked or the action being requested.

Table 2.8. Multiple Choice Checklist

Count	Revised Bloom's Taxonomy	Action	Question
	Creating Putting together ideas or elements to develop an original idea or engage in creative thinking	Constructing Designing Devising Planning Producing	• Can you design a...to...? • Can you see a possible solution to...? • If you had access to all resources, how would you deal with...? • Why don't you devise your own way to...? • What would happen if ...? • How many ways can you...? • Can you create new and unusual uses for...?
	Evaluating Judging the value of ideas, materials, and methods by developing and applying standards and criteria	Checking Critiquing Detecting Hypothesizing Judging Testing	• What are the consequences...? • Does a influence b? • What are the pros and cons of...? • What is the connection? • What are the alternatives? • Who will gain & who will lose? • What do you think will happen?
	Analyzing Breaking information down into its component elements	Attributing Comparing Deconstructing Integrating Organizing Outlining Structuring	• Did you expect certain events to occur? If not, why not? • What might be a different ending? • How is...similar to...? • What do you see as other possible outcomes? • What structure did you see in both elements? What was different?
	Applying	Carrying out Executing Implementing Using	• Do you know of another situation where this may occur? • How does this apply to real life? • Can you group by critical elements such as...? • Which factors would you change if you could and why? • What questions would you ask yourself?
	Understanding Understanding of given information	Classifying Comparing Exemplifying Explaining Inferring Interpreting Paraphrasing Summarizing	• Paraphrase this chapter in the book. • Retell in your own words. • Outline the main points. • Write a brief outline to explain this story to someone else. • Explain why the character solved the problem in this particular way.
	Remembering Recall or recognition of specific information	Describing Finding Identifying Listing Locating Naming Recognizing Retrieving	• What happened after...? • How many...? • What is...? • Who was it that...? • Name the...? • Find the definition of... • Describe what happened after... • Who did x...? • List facts that you found

Reflection:

Assessment checklist: Constructed–Response Items

	Is the assessment standards based?
	Is the level of the question comparable to a multiple-choice question? If the level is similar to a multiple-choice question, should it be offered as multiple-choice with a different question posed?
	Are clear directions provided so students will know what to do?
	If prompts are provided, are they clear so that a specific answer is needed or is the prompt ambiguous and many answers can be correct?
	Does your prompt contain a grammatical clue? For example, if your prompt asks for an, then the choice will begin with a vowel.
	Is your prompt concise?
	How many choices are you planning?
	Do you have a scoring guide for the answer key?
	Will exemplars be provided with the answer key so students will know the critical elements of each point so they can self-regulate their leaning?
	As you review the kinds of question being asked, will the answers provide data to you on what the students have learned?
	Is the assessment going to be for learning or of learning?

Reflection

Assessments for Learning

If the intent of teaching is to get students to think, the intent of formative assessment is for the teacher to understand the student's thinking.

Formative assessments should help determine what the students have mastered, what they still need, and what needs to happen next. Formative assessments are ongoing assessments, reviews, and observations in a classroom. Teachers use formative assessment to improve instructional methods and provide student feedback throughout the teaching and learning process.

Formative assessments are ongoing assessments, reviews, and observations in a classroom. Teachers should think of formative assessments as a tool to improve instructional methods and provide student feedback throughout the teaching and learning process. It is a rich source of information.

Teachers should separate the two ways in which assessments can be used. Formative assessments can be used for instructional planning (for learning) and for instructional delivery (of learning). The assessments provide teachers with feedback regarding how the students are grasping the concepts. Based on the feedback, the teacher can monitor and adjust the lesson delivery and tailor subsequent instruction based on individual student feedback.

Teachers should remember that the primary purpose of standards-based classroom assessment is to inform the instruction so as to improve learning. Classroom assessment is much more than the teacher delivering the plan lesson without checking to determine if the students understand the material. More importantly, the data should be shared with students so they can manage and monitor their learning. Testing and assessments become their friends and not their foes.

Table 2.9. Assessments for Learning or Assessment of Learning?

Assessment for Learning	Assessment of Learning
Will the assessment be done throughout the unit of study and not at the end so the lesson can be monitored?	Is the assessment summative or a final test?
Is the assessment different from a check for understanding? A check for understanding is done frequently thoughout the lesson.	
Is the assessment tied to standards with the understanding that there may be an overlap of the standards?	Is the assessment assessing one standard or many standards?
Will rubrics be provided so students can self-regulate their learning?	
Can students use the feedback from the assessment to build upon for future lessons?	Is it a final test? What did I learn from the results? What will I keep and what will I revise?
Will rubrics and exemplars be provided so students can use the assessment results and rubrics to improve?	What will be done with the results?
Can students use the assessment to plan a course of study for future lessons?	
Will subsequent assessments be given or is this the last one?	

Using Check for Understanding Prior to Using Assessments

Various ways to check for understanding can include doing it overtly or covertly, individually or collectively. For checking for understanding to be overt, the teacher will employ several methods to gather information whether the student is a preferred visual, auditory, or tactile learner. For the visual learner, the student may draw something, use a concept map, complete a Venn diagram, or use portable whiteboards.

Using pictures, graphs, or drawings that the students develop helps them to synthesize information that they are learning and then graphically represent what you have learned to teach.

For the tactile learner, students prefer to take notes during the instruction and share the information with the teacher using whiteboards, highlighting specific passages or making a list of keywords from their notes.

For the auditory learner, strategies can include turn and talk, pair-share, working in a small group to discuss their findings then sharing that information with the rest of the class. At the end of this chapter there is a chart listing some of these interventions.

Using Assessments for Lesson Planning and Shifting the Student Mindset

Assessments, in order to be useful to the teacher for lesson planning, begin with the establishment of long- and short-term goals. The short-term goal is the Student Learning Target (objective) that identifies what the student must know. The Demonstration of Student Learning (DSL) is an assessment wherein the student can demonstrate to the teacher what they know by providing evidence. The student will demonstrate to the teacher that he or she can apply what was taught. The focus of learning is a shift for the student from being a consumer (taking the learning in) to a producer (applying what was learned). The mental shift is from: what I am doing during a lesson to what I will be doing after the lesson: the shift from learning the skill (a learning activity) to applying the skill (learning outcome.) This mindset shift that the role of assessment plays is extremely important.

Shift from School Dependent to Self-Dependent

The "self-dependent learner" becomes the self-dependent learner by promoting a self-regulation learner. The shift is from an instructional focus on what must be taught to a focus on having students apply what is taught. By understanding the student's culture, language, and cognition, it builds in a schema whereby the student feels connected to the learning. That process helps the student make connections and use their prior knowledge and experiences for the new learning. That process is the forethought stage.

The Forethought Stage is the first stage of the process. The next phase is for the student to monitor and regulate their learning. (*Regulation*)

The student does not have to wait for the teacher to direct, guide, or tell them how to think but instead must become self-regulated. The shift toward self-regulation begins with teaching students self-regulation strategies. The teacher begins the process by the use of formative assessments to differentiate the student's learning then having the student be accountable for her learning by self-monitoring and self-managing the learning.

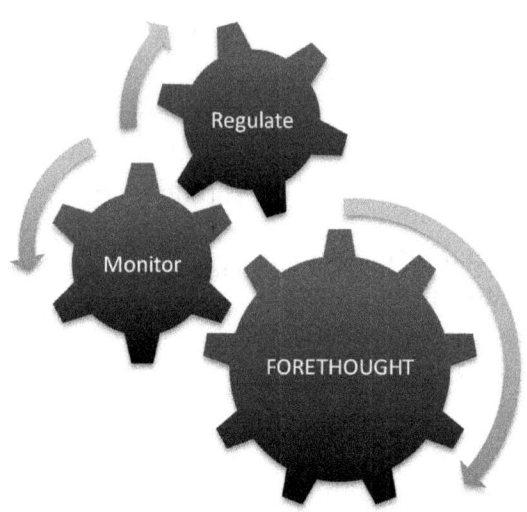

Self-Regulation Strategies

How-to instruction for Self-Regulated Learning Strategies
Effective instructional practices for helping students learn self-regulation are:
1. Develop and promote student self-efficacy • Support learners to believe in themselves. • Promote effort as opposed to attribution. Smart is not what you are but what you can be. • Help students set goals and promote high expectations. Reach for the stars. • Promote a growth mindset and not a fixed mindset. The key word is "yet": You may not have gotten the work correct yet but it will come. • Frame new information or feedback in a positive rather than a negative manner (e.g., "keeping track of your homework assignments will help you manage this course successfully," rather than "if you don't keep track you will fail"). • Provide specific cues for using self-regulatory strategies. After the cues are provided, have students start to incorporate the strategies into their daily routines. • Remember: Self-regulation skills must be taught
2. Promote reflective dialogue • Have students practice "oral rehearsals" • Model reflective practices (thinking aloud) so students will understand the strategy. Practice an example by talking through the process so student will hear the thought process to use when they are doing the problem. • Ask reflective questions to promote reflective dialogue. Have students share their reflections with a partner. • Use the power of groups to promote robust discussions to think through problems/cases (collaborative learning). • Have students ask "why" questions to seek deeper understandings. • Promote application of concepts rather that knowing facts.
3. Provide feedback • Provide feedback based on standards or rubrics so students know the feedback is not personal, biased, or based on prejudice. • Use standards to show students what the next level is for them to achieve. • Feedback should be specific, focused, and timely. Students should use the feedback to refine their approach and reshape their thinking. • Base feedback (positive or constructive) on the task, not on the learner.
4. Help learners make connections between abstract concepts • Abstract concepts are hard to understand so multiple approaches must be used, for example, visual, manipulatives, graphics. • Provide hands-on learning activities. • Provide factual information with the abstract so students see connection. • Have students discuss ideas to promote metacognition
5. Help learners link new experiences to prior learning to promote "bridging" stored knowledge with new knowledge • Use a Readiness set to begin the process of "bridging." • Help students see connections by using experiential learning activities. • Focus on application so students see the value of what they are learning.

There are now two important considerations for the teacher to be mindful throughout the lesson: one, to do frequent checks of understanding and/or other formative assessments; and two, give feedback to students that will be timely, constructive, and encouraging so as to promote student success.

The failure to provide feedback or have limited feedback during the lesson does not provide guidance for the student and the student may presume that she is doing well. Additionally, feedback is needed to encourage students to continue to try. Actually, it has been my experience that students who are not given any feedback during a lesson or after doing a task, tend to rate themselves higher on their achievement.

Although teachers want to encourage students so they continue to try hard, students need feedback to ensure they are progressing properly. It is the feedback that enables the student to assess how well they are doing on a test.

Stress Attribution

Encouraging students to do well is one aspect of "attribution theory." Attribution theory postulates that the manner in which students explain or "attribute" failure and/or success is based on their ability, for example, I am smart so I will do well. How many times have you heard students say: "I wasn't lucky today; the test was too hard; I need to study better next time," etc. The other attributes include the ability, will, and the difficulty of the task.

Of all the attributes, encouraging effort provides the most effective results. Promoting effort is effective because:

1. If students believe that failure was a result of lack of trying, they are more likely to remain optimistic about trying in the future. How many times have teachers told students to "try harder."
2. *Hard work pays off* is an adage for students so they believe more effort is needed and will not feel "stupid" or that they lack capacity.
3. When teachers encourage students to try harder and they succeed from trying hard, they will feel better about themselves and take pride in what they have accomplished. The feeling of pride will offset the guilt they feel if they fail.

It's not unusual to see elementary teachers give stickers or prizes to students who try hard during an activity. Additionally, teachers will also give students words of encouragement to help them try harder on the next assignment. Intuitively, teachers are encouraging students to continue to try hard so they will become successful and feel good about what they have accomplished as a result of their effort.

What are some other ways for assessments to help students?

Cognitive Strategies in Enhancing Learning

Three general principles that are very inexpensive to employ and enhance cognitive strategies to improve student learning are:

1. Have students understand the concept of "distribution" (spacing and interleaving) of material and practice during learning. When to study and how to study is important for self-regulation and self-modulation of learning.
2. Encourage frequent assessment of learning (direct and indirect positive effects of quizzing and testing). The assessments can be part of their distribution schedule. For example, during massed practice, I will assess myself after every chapter.
3. Encourage students to use explanatory questioning (elaborate interrogation and self-explanation) as a way to promote sense and meaning.

Table 2.11. Elaborative Interrogation Form

Notes from the reading
This make sense because: (Answer why the material makes sense)

Let's see how the three principles can be applied to assessment beginning with distributed practice or "distribution."

Distribution addresses the concept of spacing and interleaving material as well as being a strategy to use during learning. Distribution can also be practiced as a learning strategy for the student to use while doing home learning.

The general notion is that practice makes perfect, as exemplified by students continually practicing a task. An example would be to practice the multiplication times tables numerous times by writing them over and over so it helps the student memorize the facts. The practice of repeating a task over and over again is one way to learn and is referred to as mass or blocked practice.

The other way to learn information would be to space the practice or distribute the practice over time. Using the process of distribution, the information is spaced over time. The effects of spacing material are effective over a period of time as opposed to studying the day or night before a test, which is known as cramming.

Cramming before a test can result in short-term success; however, it will not be held in memory for a long period of time. Cramming and rushing through readings are not ideal ways to feel ready for any academic challenge. I would often tell my students that all the caffeine and energy drink in the world to stay up the night before a test is not the best way to study for long-term memory or retention as it does not make effective use of time or develop effective study habits for self-regulation.

Who among us has not studied the night before a test and actually did well on the test? And if you did do well, how did you feel after the test?

One effective way to study would be to space the learning over time. That practice is "spacing."

The teacher can also apply spacing concept during the period of instructional delivery. It is the concept of "prime time/downtime and primary/recent." Prime time/downtime and primacy/recency was written about by Sousa (2000, 2001). He based his work on the research done by Ebbinghaus (1885).

The basic premise is that students will remember information that is covered at the beginning of a class period, which is referred to as prime time. Students will also remember information that is presented at the end of a period, which is referred to as recency.

If information is introduced at the beginning of a class period (prime time A), students can work on it for a period of time (downtime), while the last part of the class period can be used for prime time again (prime time B). During the "downtime" activity, teachers can assess student progress.

As the assessments are done, the teacher can establish skill groups based on the targeted instruction during the independent learning time or during guided practice. It is during the guided practice that the teacher questions the student to determine the depth of the student's knowledge regarding their understanding what must be done. The teacher can also encourage the student to self-monitor or self-regulate their learning. Another approach to help students learn is to use interleaving.

SUMMARY

1. Use massed practice or distributed strategies for learning.
2. Use interleaving with problem-solving activities.
3. Use multi-modal strategies like combing graphics with verbal descriptors.
4. Connect concrete representations when presenting abstract concepts.
5. Use assessments for learning as well as of learning.
6. Spacing can be massed or distributed. Have students understand when to use massed or distributed practice and plan accordingly.
7. Encourage students to remember that growth is a process, so if they do not do well initially, they can revise their study habits. Remember: You are not there "yet" but you will be.

Table 2.12. Spacing Plan for Test Study

(Test is a week away) Date of test: Study protocols: notes, partners, review, memorize facts, write out definitions, elaborative interrogation, other	Practice: Study one week before the test Date one week before test: Reflection:
	Study the night before the test Date
(Test is a month away) Date of test Study protocols: notes, partners, review, memorize facts, write out definitions, elaborative interrogation, other	Study four weeks before the test Study date Study protocols used
	Study a week before the test Study date Study protocols used
	Review day before the test:
(Test is six months away) Date of test Study protocols: notes, partners, review, memorize facts, write out definitions, elaborative interrogation, other	Study five months before the test Study date Study protocols used
	Study three months before the test Study date Study protocols used
	Study week before the test: Date
	Review day before the test:

Implementing Interleaving

An example of implementing interleaving would be to have the students do four examples. One example is worked out for the students with an explanation of the process used to get the answer. In this manner, the student will see how to solve the problem and the thinking process used so they can start the process of self-regulation. The problem with its answer is "interleaved" amongst the other problems.

The teacher can also use interleaving in the classroom during student independent work time. One way for this to occur would be for students to present the answers to their tablemate. After the students spend X amount of time working on their project, they can turn to their neighbor to explain what they have done. The tablemate will have answers to the problems that were assigned and check to see if the student did the work correctly.

The interleaving allows students to self-regulate their learning as they see the answer and use that knowledge to modulate and monitor their own learning. The correct answer can also serve as an example for the student in solving the problem and the thought process involved in its resolution.

Other Ways to Promote Self-Regulation

One strategy would be for the teacher to call upon a student to explain their process to someone at their table. Classmates can assess the student explanation. This format can be problematic as only one student is doing the work while the remaining students are checking that work. It is much more desirable to have students work in pairs so that they are involved in more of the discussion.

Another approach to formative assessments would be student driven and involves the use of self-explanation and elaborative interrogation. With elaborative interrogation, the student will ask why the fact was stated; a defensible explanation is required for the answer. The purpose of this activity is to ensure that the student begins to develop a deeper understanding why something is occurring and can articulate the reasons for her answer.

Having students explain their thinking process when they are doing an assignment can be helpful. Students can also justify why they use various methods. This is one form of oral rehearsal.

In both cases, the role of the teacher would be to question students to determine how well they can explain what they are doing. The important consideration is that students are beginning to develop metacognition as well as self-regulation.

A critical point to remember is that the teacher needs to be aware of the student's thinking to ensure that she is proceeding appropriately. The monitoring can be done during the lesson and/or during a student conference. If the teacher has a large class, she can also have the students keep a journal and review the journals during the class period or after the class period.

Another method of formative assessments is quizzes. A quick quiz given during a lesson will provide feedback to the teacher on what information the student has obtained and what needs to be taught. Assessments can have a positive effect on student achievement as the teacher will know what students have learned and what points remain troublesome.

Roediger and Pye also site research in which frequent assessments of 5 to 10 minutes produces a large game performance (Leming, 2002; Lyle and Cranford, 2011; in Roediger and Pye, 2012).

Student self-testing and quizzes will prompt the students to use tests/quizzes for learning and not just assessments. Students will quickly realize that self-testing will enable them to see what they need to study, what they understand, what the next steps are for more effective comprehension.

In the next chapter we look at closing a lesson.

Important Points

The question therefore is what do effective teachers do?

1. Effective teachers have well-planned lessons that start with an objective and an essential question
2. Maintain effective classroom management
3. Communicate learning goals
4. Plan cooperative activities, practice skills using activities
5. Use of quizzes for learning
6. Have high student involvement
7. Use formative assessments to improve learning
8. Teach self-regulation skills
9. Use assessment of learning and for learning

REFERENCES

Allen, J., and Gregory, Anne, Mikami, Amori, Lun, Janetta, Hamre, Bridget, and Pianta, Robert. (March 2013). Observations of effective teacher-student interactions in secondary school classrooms: Predicting student achievement with classroom assessment scoring system. *School Psychology Review 42* (1).

Black, P., and Uilian, D. (1998). Assessment and Classroom Learning. School of Education, King's College London.

Black, P., and Wiliam, D. (1998). Inside the Black Box: Raising Standards Through Classroom Assessment. British Education Research Association, Phi Delta Kappan, 139–144, 146–148.

Bjork, R. (1994). Memory and metamemory considerations in training of human beings. In J. Metcalfe and A. Shimamura (eds.), *Metacognition: Knowing about Learning*. Cambridge, MA: MIT Press, pp. 185–205.

Dufour, Richard et al. (2004). Whatever It Takes: How Professional Learning Communities Respond When Kids Don't Learn, Bloomington, Ind.: National Educational Service

Hattie, J. A. (1992). Do teachers count? *Australian Association for Pastoral Care in Education 2*, 9–11.

Hattie, J. A. (1992). Towards a model of schooling: A synthesis of meta-analyses. *Australian Journal of Education 36*, 5–13.

Dufour, Richard et al. (2004). *Whatever It Takes: How Professional Learning Communities Respond When Kids Don't Learn*. Bloomington, IN: National Educational Service.

Hattie, J. A. (1992). Do teachers count? *Australian Association for Pastoral Care in Education*, *2*, 9–11.

Hattie, J. A. (1992). Towards a model of schooling: A synthesis of meta-analyses. *Australian Journal of Education*, *36*, 5–13.

Leming, F. C. (2002). The exam-a-day procedure improves performance in psychology classes. *Teaching of Psychology 29* (3), 210–212.

Lyle, K. B., and Crawford, N. A. (2011). Retrieving essential material at the end of lectures improves performance on statistics exams. *Teaching of Psychology 38*, 94–97.

Marzano, Robert. (2006). *Classroom Assessment and Grading That Work*. Alexandria, VA: Association for Supervision and Curriculum Development.

Marzano, R., Marzano, J., and Pickering, D. (2003). *Classroom Management That Works: Research-Based Strategies for Every Teacher*. Alexandria, VA: Association for Supervision and Curriculum Development.

Marzano, R., Pickering, D., and Pollock, J. (2001). *Classroom Instruction That Works: Research-Based Strategies for Increasing Student Achievement*. Alexandria, VA: Association for Supervision and Curriculum Development.

Roediger, H., and Pye, M. A. (2012). Applying cognitive psychology to education: Complexities and prospects. *Journal of Applied Research in Memory & Cognition, 1*(4), 263–265.

Roediger, H., and Pye, M. A., (2012). Inexpensive techniques to improve education: Applying cognitive psychology to enhance educational practice. *Journal of Applied Research in Memory & Cognition, 1*, 242–248.

Sousa, David (2000). *How the Brain Learns*. Thousand Oaks, CA: Corwin Press.

Sousa, David (2001). *How the Brain Learns, Second Edition*. Thousand Oaks, CA: Corwin Press.

Wright, S. P., Horn, S., and Sanders, W. (1997). Teacher and classroom context effects n student achievement: Implications for teacher evaluation. *Journal of Personnel Evaluation in Education* (11), 57– 67. Retrieved December 6, 2007, from http://www.sas.com/govedu/edu/teacher_eval.pdf

3

Closing Stage of the Learner's Brain Model

Consolidation for Closure

FOCUS OF THE CHAPTER

The teacher will learn strategies to use for Consolidation for Closure. The teacher will also be able to show the students strategies they can use for self-regulation when doing home learning.

INTRODUCTION

Consolidation for Closure is a process whereby the learner will summarize what has been learned. Although closure is usually done at the end of a lesson, it can be done during the lesson. What research says about closure will be provided and overt or covert closure strategies for visual, auditory, tactile or kinesthetic learners.

PROBING QUESTIONS

1. Why is Consolidation for Closure done?
2. How will the student show the teacher what they learned?
3. How will the teacher use what the students learned to plan tomorrow's lesson?
4. Can overt or cover Consolidation for Closure use visual, auditory, kinetics, or tactile strategies?

BACKGROUND

In the Learner's Brain Model, the final stage of the lesson is Consolidation for Closure. The Learner's Brain Model provides a model to help focus classroom teachers by getting information from the student, facilitating student practice with guidance, and subsequently offering independent practice to solidify the learning. In the appendix there are rubrics that can be used for coaching.

CONSOLIDATION FOR CLOSURE IS THE FINAL STEP OF THE LEARNER'S BRAIN MODEL

The process is called Consolidation for Closure. The purpose is for students to consolidate the information they learned during the lesson and articulate to the teacher what they are consolidating, for example, "Today I learned . . ." The information tells the teacher how the student processed the lesson. This is extremely important information as the brain consolidates information when the student sleeps.

The teacher would want the correct information to be processed and saved while the student sleeps. Since consolidation is the last step of the teacher's lesson, it is important that the teacher is aware of what the student takes away from the lesson.

With overt closure, the student tells the teacher what she learned today. In this process, it is obvious what the student feels is important. This task is a little more difficult with covert closure as the student is writing what she has learned. The teacher may not see the comments until after the student leaves and is given an exit ticket. The teacher will have to follow up with the student the next day and the exit ticket becomes an "entrance ticket' as it begins the discussion in the next class.

CONSOLIDATION FOR CLOSURE

This process is the last step in a lesson and is a valuable tool. Unfortunately, it is an essential lesson plan element that many times is overlooked and skipped. It often receives "short shrift" for a variety of reasons. Many teachers claim it is because there is just not enough time to cover everything they want to teach. Another reason closure is not done is that teachers think that review is a closure activity.

In some cases Consolidation for Closure is not done as the teacher gets involved in the lesson and teaches until the bell rings or until the end of the period. Teachers may believe that they have to teach "bell to bell" so they do not want to spend time at the end of the period doing a closure activity.

Below are a few examples of Covert Closure that a teacher can use. There is also Overt Closure that can be done and examples will be provided.

Overt	
Tell a Friend;	Students work in pairs and share what they learned. They consult and report their finding to the teacher.
I have an answer, who has a question?	Students write a question in which the answer captures the critical component of what they learned. Teacher collects the questions to use as a review for the next day's lesson. (A Readiness Set).
We be three	Students work in teams of three and share what they learned. A spokesperson is selected for the group and they share what was discussed. The rest to the class gives a thumbs up or thumbs down if they agree or disagree.
Thesis Statement:	Students summarize what they learn and then consolidate the information into a thesis statement
Today and tomorrow	For Today: Students write on an index card what they learned from the lesson. They also list key talk away points. For Tomorrow: Students write how the information applies for future lessons.
Writing Conference:	Students are given three questions to answer then pair-share with a buddy what they learned. They summarize what they learned and share it with the class. The student selects one key point to write about at home.
Response Logs:	Student write in their response log what they believe is the critical elements of the lesson. The teacher reviews the logs and gives the students feedback.
Student Checklist:	Teacher has several questions she asks the students and their answers are noted on a checklist
Give Me Three	Students summarize what they learn in 3 sentences.
Strikeout	Students write three key points from the lesson: Strike 1, 2 and 3
Now What?	Students share how the information applies to the real world
Beat The Clock	Students are given 30 seconds to think about what they learned. The teacher calls on students to share what they learned in 30 seconds. After the first round, students and given 30 seconds to think about what they heard and will be given 30 seconds for a round two. For Round 2, students can not repeat what was previously stated.
My Student Learning Target	Students write the Student Learning Target and a short summary of what they learned and how it supports the Learning Target. "Today I learned x, and it is tied to the Student Learning Target by y."
Stand out	Something that stands out form today's lesson is......

Overt Closure Examples

News Headline	News Headline: Students write a "Headline" for a newspaper. Students write a paragraph about their Headline
Write a test question	Students write a test question based on what they learned. Teacher will collect all the questions and use them to develop a quiz. The test questions will provide teacher information on what seems important.
Overt	
Connect the dots	Students add to what was previously stated and justify their addition.
Pick a partner	Students pick – clock partners (Everyone is assigned d a time, i.e., 1:00, 2:00 etc. All the 1:00 meet, all the 2:00 meet) Football or baseball buddies. Students pick their favorite teams. Job buddies – students who want to pursue the same profession. Students pick a partner and discuss what they learned then share their findings.
Explain and predict	Students explain one thing they learned and predict how it can be applied.
Create a Brochure	Students design a brochure which illustrate main points of what they learned and use it as an entrance ticket for the next day's class.
My Turn, Your Turn, Share	I talk, you talk then we develop a message for the teacher
Salt shaker	List key points (salt) from today's lesson
Rowboat	Students write key points to put in the rowboat

Covert	
Look inside	Students write a letter to their parents about what they learned today.
Challenge question	Students write a a challenge question based on whath they laerned and post it to their class account. The next day the teacher selects a question for the class to answer. Since the calss does not know what question will be used, they have to review the total lsit of questions for home learning tto b eprepared for the class "quiz" the next day.
Next step	Students will describe what they will do with the information they learned. For example, I learned x and it is needed to do y. Fact → Concept → Application
Lesson Salesperson	Students write a "sales pitch" on how to use what they learned in class.
Math Talk	Student discusses the Mathematical Practices that were used in the lesson. They talk about what they learned, how it applies and the reasoning or mathematical mindset taught.
Use a Graphic Organizer to show Cause and effect	CAUSE • EFFECT • EFFECT → CAUSE • EFFECT • EFFECT
	EFFECT / CAUSE / EVENT CAUSE — ☐ EFFECT ☐ EFFECT ☐ EFFECT CAUSE — ☐ EFFECT ☐ EFFECT ☐ EFFECT

Thought Bubble (Social Studies). Select an event or a person and describe that they might be thinking about an event; think about next steps.	
Comic Strip Students develop a comic strip of what they learned	
Timeline	
Point-Counter point	Show two different perspectives by making a point and developing a counter point. Use talk bubble Dr Martin Luther King Malcolm X

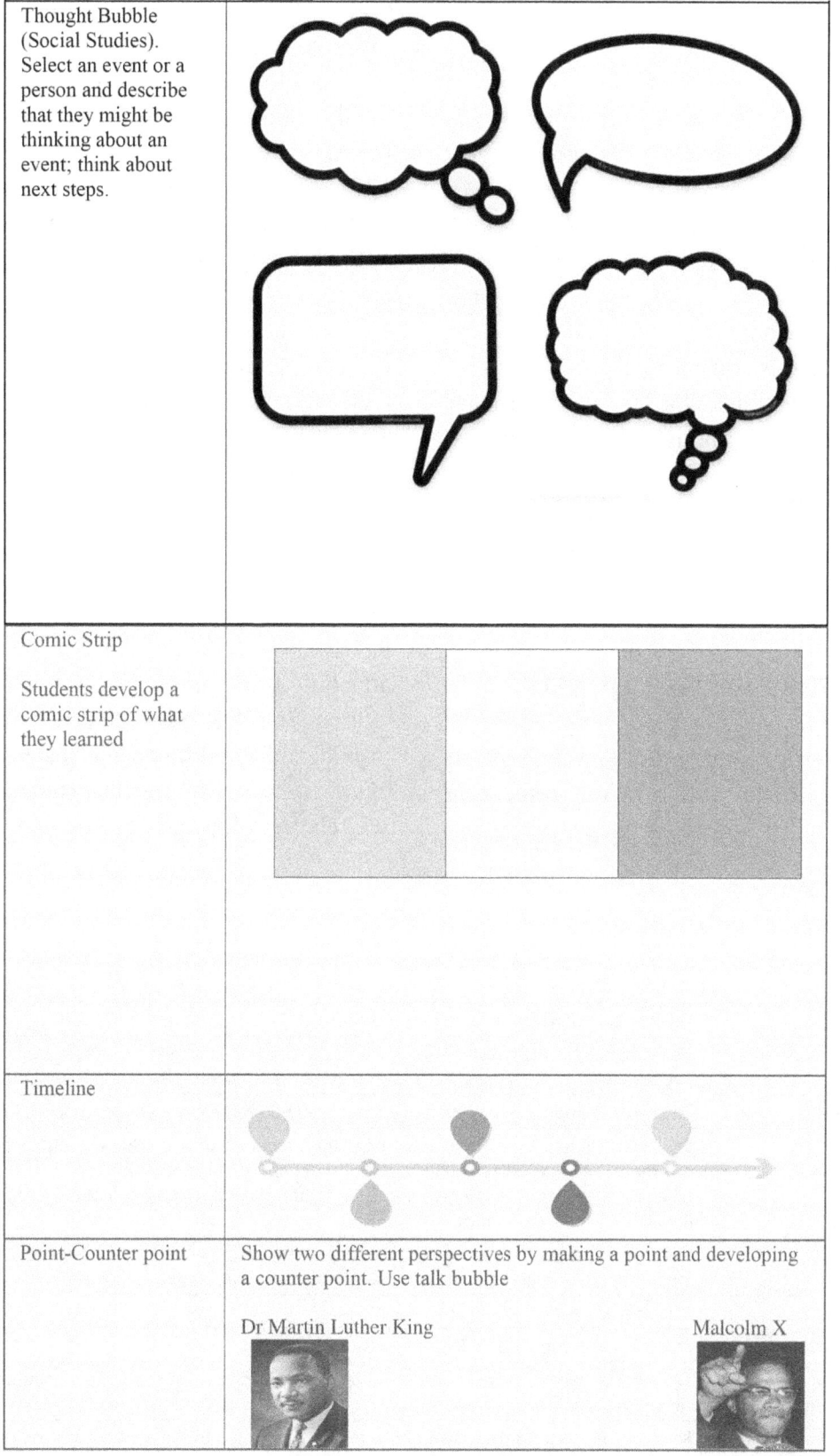

REVIEW OR CLOSURE

In some teachers' minds, a review is closure. When a review is done, however, it is usually the teacher who is doing the talking. "Do you remember, class, we talked about X?" Or the teacher may say, "Remember, we covered X last week." Unfortunately, the process of the teacher talking is not closure as it is the student who must do the talking in a closure activity.

When the teacher is doing the talking during a review, she is summarizing of the lesson. The teacher uses that opportunity to bring together her ideas. A quick rule of thumb is: If the teacher talks, it is review; if the student talks it is closure. Remember, the goal is for the student to talk and share her ideas so as to consolidate the information.

CLOSURE BACKGROUND

Closure is a term from gestalt psychology. It refers to an automatic process in our perception where we "close" incomplete figures, where we "connect the dots" or fill in the gaps. A classic example is a picture of three dots in a straight line. We tend to see a line, not three separate dots. If the three dots are in the shape of a triangle, we see the triangle, not the separate dots.

One applies the psychological process of closure when looking at the three dots whether they are in a straight line or in the shape of a triangle and form a whole, or gestalt, out of the three dots.

Since the brain is a "pattern seeker" and looks for completeness, when closure is blocked, one feels anxiety and is motivated to try to reduce that anxiety. The mind likes to form wholes, gestalts. We like to see a complete big picture. When this process is blocked, the brain will fill in the blanks to make it complete.

Closure is also an important process for the learner because the learner will summarize what has been learned and engage in the process of attaching sense and meaning to the learned information. The talk and summary by the student will provide information to the teacher who can ask clarifying questions to the student to help them see relationships and develop understanding.

Table 3.1. Review or What Closure Is NOT

Review	What closure IS NOT
Teacher summarizes the lesson	Teacher tells the class: Does everyone remember? Today we talked about X. Here are some facts you should know.
Teacher talk	Teacher summarizes the lesson for the student.
Does anyone have a question?	Does anyone have a question? Teacher asks a question and then answers her own question. The teacher accepts silence as an answer to her question as there are no questions.
Teacher validation	Today we learned X. Does everyone agree? Do you remember we talked about X?
Fact value	Students state a fact and the teacher takes the statement at face value without clarifying the comment. This is especially critical if a misconception is stated. Once the statement is made, the task is to go to the next person and not get answers but to move the activity along to get it done.
Teacher activity	Students do an activity to end the class period. For example, students complete a worksheet during the closure period and are asked to complete the task at home.
"Rate my lesson"	Students rate a teacher's lesson.
Home learning activity	Students are given a home learning assignment to do.
Using closed questions instead of open questions	Teacher has several closed questions—yes or no questions—with the goal being to see how many students agree.
"Pack up and get ready to leave"	Students are asked to pack their books to get ready to go to the next class. While students are packing, the teacher reviews her lesson.
Playing a game	Students play a game that has entertainment value but no educational value.

WHAT DOES RESEARCH SAY ABOUT CLOSURE?

Marzano's research on instructional design states that setting objectives and providing feedback, specifically asking students to assess themselves at the end of a unit "will yield a 23 percent gain" (Marzano, Pinkering, and Pollock, 2001, p. 83).

When a teacher asks clarifying questions to a student at the end of a lesson, the purpose of the questioning is to help the student reframe their thinking and/or look at their thinking with fresh eyes. What is even more interesting is the research done by Restak (2006) in which he describes the process of "backward framing."

Restak states that backward framing design alters an already established memory. The definition that he cites is taken from Gerald Zaltman's text: "How customers think: what consumers recall about prior products or shopping experiences will differ from their actual experiences if marketers refer to those past experiences in a positive way" (Restak, 2006, p. 160).

The research claimed that consumers can be influenced to recall their prior experiences differently; in essence, their thinking can be reconstructed. Keeping this principle in mind, closure can be very important as the teacher uses the process during "overt closure" and ask students questions to help them clarify their thinking. Or the teacher can use the information gathered from the students from "covert closure" to plan new lessons that will focus on developing accurate and deliberate information.

Table 3.2. Closure versus Checking for Understanding (CFU)

Closure	Checking for Understanding
A formative assessment used at the end of a lesson.	Checks for Understanding (CFU) can be done: ✓ Visual performance check: Students provide a visual sign to the instructor, for example, thumbs up, down, or sideways. ✓ Auditory
A planned strategy after a lesson is taught. Closure	Teacher questions students throughout the lesson to determine the pacing of the lesson and student knowledge. CFU
Overt or Covert	Can be done overtly and covertly
Closure is done at the end of a lesson. Adjustments to the learning are done after the closure activity, which is normally at the end of a class period.	CFU are done while the lesson is being taught. Real-time adjustments are made during the instructional delivery.
Closure can also be done using visual, auditory, or tactile venues.	CFU can be done visually, auditorily, or tactilely.
Closure is done after the lesson so it will not affect the pace to the lesson unless the teacher reteaches the lesson based on the information gathered from closure.	CFU help to pace a lesson
Backbone of planning as information is collected and used for subsequent lessons.	Backbone of Explicit Direct Instruction
Closure is done after the teaching is done.	Teaching is done first, so teachers present the content then check for understanding.
Used for teacher planning.	Used for student planning: ensures that students will not practice their home learning incorrectly.
Closure asks one basic question: What did you learn today?	CFU use teacher questions to gather information. Based on the answers given, the teacher can determine if students are ready to move on.
Summative assessment of a lesson to evaluate the lesson according to the Student Learning Target.	Formative assessment: frequent, interactive checking of student progress to identify student learning needs for the teacher to make lesson adjustments.

CLOSURE TECHNIQUES: BACKWARD FRAMING

The technique of applying "backward framing" to Consolidation for Closure would start by taking the information gathered by the teacher from the student and use it as a frame of reference of what needs to be addressed. The teacher can then plan the new lesson with the information gained by tying in the information that was previously discussed. The new lesson will introduce new bits of information, facts, data, etc., that was not discussed in a previous lesson.

The introduction of the new material would begin the process of backward framing or having the students view the information through a different lens. After the new information is presented, the teacher can have discussions with the students about the new bits of information.

Restak wrote about an example of backward framing done by Kathryn Braun in which unsuspecting subjects were shown an advertisement for Disney. The ad suggested that children visiting Disneyland would shake hands with Bugs Bunny (people who know Disney know that Bugs Bunny is a Warner Bros. creation and not a Disney creation). Interestingly enough about 16 percent of adults who read the ad recalled meeting Bugs Bunny during a childhood visit to Disneyland! On the contrary, those who did not read the ad did not recall meeting Bugs Bunny (Restak, 2006). The power of suggestion is very strong.

CONSOLIDATION FOR CLOSURE PROCESS

The critical attribute of Consolidation for Closure is that it is a process whereby the learner will summarize what has been learned. The student will have had time to practice and rehearse what was taught and attach sense and meaning to it. The talk and summary by the student will provide information to the teacher.

Although closure is usually done at the end of a lesson, there are various times it can be done. Specifically:

- It can be done at the beginning of a lesson to summarize the previous day's assignment and develop readiness for the new lesson.
- Unlike a "Readiness Set" which is also done at the beginning of a lesson to develop student readiness by activating prior knowledge, this activity is directly related to the previous day's lesson. For example: "Class, yesterday we talked about the Revolutionary War and you had an assignment to do for home learning."
- Be prepared to discuss two facts from the lesson or your homework assignment.

PROCEDURAL CLOSURE

Procedural closure can occur during the lesson (called procedural closure) when the teacher moves from one objective to the next. As the teacher is reviewing an activity in a lesson that involves procedural tasks, the teacher will do a procedural closure. This practice is common in math as students are doing procedural activities and the teacher is seeking feedback from the students.

The process begins with the teacher asking the class to pair-share with their table mates the rules of operation that was discussed. After the discussion, the teacher asks the students to apply the rules of operation to the new problems. During the share out, students should have a print-out of the rules to ensure that they are stating the proper rules.

CONSOLIDATION CLOSURE AT THE END OF THE LESSON

Closure at the end of a lesson is called consolidation closure. The purpose is to ensure that students are leaving with the correct information and that is why it is called closure for consolidation. The process begins again with the planning stage based upon student information. The circle is complete.

CLOSURE BENEFITS

Lesson closure has many benefits which is why teachers need to set time aside for a consolidation for closure activity. It is important for a teacher to set aside a short, concentrated time period of approximately six to eight minutes for closure whenever closure is done. This is a time for students to put together everything they learned and make sense out of what has just been taught. The teacher simply asking, "Does anyone have any questions?" and students answering, "No" is not closure. This process does not provide feedback to the teacher which is needed if closure is to be effective.

Closure provides important feedback for both the teacher and the student. During closure, the activity assigned to the student by the teacher provides the teacher feedback about the lesson taught. It will give the teacher an idea if additional practice time is needed, if the lesson needs to be retaught, or if it is okay to move on to the next concept. After closure, if the objective was mastered, the teacher can then make the decision to move on to a new objective. Consequently, if teachers are not making time for this important element in the lesson planning and lesson delivery, it is difficult to gauge if students understood the material and have mastered the concepts and skills set at the beginning of the lesson.

Some argue the fact that not all lesson plans should contain consolidation for closure in every single lesson plan. Closure is the exception because it is useful for the student and the teacher. Closure provides the students the opportunity to reflect. It gives them the chance to reflect and digest what was taught. It also provides the teacher with the data to determine if the desired learning outcome of the lesson was reached. The information from closure is needed to facilitate and enhance student accomplishment especially if the student did not understand what was taught. What are some examples of closure activities?

Closure Example

Some examples of closure activities include students writing a summary describing what was learned in the lesson, making a timeline plotting the events that were discussed in class, or using an exit slip.

Exit-slip activities serve as a great closure activity because they provide an easy way for the teacher to assess understanding and can be quickly completed on scrap paper or on an index card. Some teachers use the "3-2-1 strategy," whereby students write down three things that interested them, two things they learned, and one question they have.

According to Dale's Cone of Experience, we learn 10 percent of what we read, 20 percent of what we hear, 30 percent of what we see, 40 percent of what we both see and hear, 70 percent of what is discussed with others, 80 percent of what we experience personally, and 95 percent of what we teach someone else. Based on this research, teachers should remember to provide students not only the opportunities to learn, but also the opportunity to teach others. As a closing activity, one might have the students model how they solved a math equation or share how they decided on their opening sentence to their writing piece through a "think aloud" presentation.

CLOSURE ACTIVITIES

As a closing activity, one can consider using questioning techniques at the end of a lesson. One should incorporate higher-level questions, not rote recall of information questions. Using question cues is great to get meaningful answers from students. The teacher presents the question and the student is required to answer the question showing the teacher that they can assimilate the information.

Possible question cues that allow the students to reflect are: I learned X and I wonder if . . . ? Teacher: How will you apply what was taught? How would you justify . . . based on what you learned? How might you apply what you learned today? How can you explain X based on what you learned?

Another closing activity is "throwing the ball." The teacher starts off by asking a question. Students raise their hand to answer the question. The teacher throws the ball to one student. That student gets a chance to answer the question. If he or she answers it correctly, they get to ask a question and throw the ball to another classmate, who in turn will answer that question.

If the student does not answer the question correctly, then the child has to throw the ball to someone else who can answer the teacher's question. During this time, they are allowed to use their notes. This encourages students to take notes during the lesson and pay attention. Most students enjoy throwing and catching the ball; therefore, they will be more attentive during the lesson so that they can later participate in the closing activity.

Another favorite is "fishbowl." For the "fishbowl" closing activity, students write a question about the lesson on a piece of paper or index card. Then they form an inner and outer circle. Students face each other and share their question with one another and see if the other person can answer the question. If time permits, students can even rotate to a new partner.

"I have a letter" is another favorite. For the "I have a letter" closing activity, each child is given an index card and they design a postcard to their parents explaining the day's lesson. This is great for the creative students who enjoy drawing and coloring.

Another excellent example shared was the creation of an "infomercial" that explains what they learned in class that day. For students that like using technology, this is a great activity as students develop an "infomercial" based on what they learned in class.

"Create a jingle" is great for the musically inclined students. In "create a jingle" students create a jingle that explains the main idea or important facts of the lesson.

For social studies teachers, "What am I?" is an excellent activity that has students create clues or riddles about the key terms and quiz each other. This activity can be done in partnerships or as a class. This activity is great as a review for a unit or chapter test.

An effective and meaningful lesson closure is "movie review" whereby students critique the lesson as if it was a movie.

If teachers consistently use closure activities in their lessons, students will become accustomed to the process and will be better prepared to close the lesson. Due to the fact that students know that they will be expected to do a closing activity, it is more likely that students will be more actively engaged in the lesson and will take ownership of the material being taught. Below are examples of closing activities tied to learning styles.

Table 3.3. Overt/Covert Closure and Closure Based on Learning Styles

Overt	Covert
Tell Me in Your Own Words: Students are asked to paraphrase what they learned.	**Tell a Friend:** Students work in pairs and share what they learned.
Tweet: Students send a tweet to the teacher. They have to consolidate what they learned into three to five key words.	**I Have an Answer, Who Has a Question?** Students write a question in which the answer captures the critical component of what they learned.
Red Light, Green Light: For elementary students. Each desk has a red or green cup. The teacher will make a statement and those who agree turn the green cup upside down.	**Signals:** Students work in teams of three and share what they learned. A spokesperson is selected for the group and they share what was discussed. The rest of the class give a thumbs-up or thumbs-down if they agree or disagree.
Brainstorm: Students share their one takeaway from the lesson and come to consensus as to the critical elements of the lesson	**Thesis Statement:** Students summarize what they learned and then consolidate the information into a thesis statement.
Whiteboards: Students use the whiteboard to write critical points of the lesson.	**Exit Tickets:** Students write on an index card what they learned from the lesson, the key takeaway points.
Think, Pair, Share: Students work in small groups, share their information, then share it with the larger group.	**Writing Conference:** Students are given three questions to answer then pair-share with a buddy what they learned. They summarize what they learned and share it with the class. The students select one key point to write about at home.
Four Corners: Teacher writes four key points to the lesson and posts each one in a corner of the room. Students select which of the four points they like and go to that corner of the room. They develop a summary statement from their small group meeting.	**Response Logs:** Student write in their response log what they believe are the critical elements of the lesson. The teacher reviews the logs and gives the students feedback.
L & A Chart: Students write what they learned and how it can be applied.	**Student Checklist:** Teacher has several questions she asks the students and their answers are noted on a checklist.
Key Words: Students write key words from the lesson.	**Short Summary:** Students summarize what they learn in three sentences.

Visual	Auditory	Kinesthetic	Tactile
Characteristics: use visual materials, i.e., maps, pictures; write, illustrate, read, use color graphs, flowcharts	**Characteristics:** lectures, discussions, debates, create mnemonics	**Characteristics:** attend labs, take frequent breaks, move, assemble collections	**Characteristics:** use printed sources, take detailed notes, use manuals, handouts, or story starters
Use of **whiteboards** Graphic organizers Mind maps Drawing Picture The purpose is to have students express what they learned using a variety of modalities.	Inventive Dialogue: **Three "Whats"** Students respond to the following: What did you learn today? What does it mean? (How is this important? relevant? useful?) What can you do with the information? (What is the practical application of the information?)	Turn and Talk: **Come to My Side** Students are arranged in two lines facing one another. Students discuss main points of the lesson to try to convince members from the other line to come to their line. **Four Corners** The teacher has four critical points noted on paper and posts one in each of the four corners of the room. Students select a critical point and stand in the corner that has the point they support.	Student Checklist: **Quick Write Likert Scale** Students respond to teacher-generated prompts (perhaps displayed on the overhead projector or on a permanent poster in the room. The prompts are from a difficult level to an application level. 1. I can apply today's lesson in the real work... 2. Today's lesson makes sense to me because... 3. I understand today's lesson because... 4. I enjoyed today's lesson but I have some questions... 5. I found today's lesson difficult because...
Concept Map: Students are given a concept map and list the main point in the center circle.	Debate: Students develop debate question to use for a class debate.	Key Word List: Students share their ideas and make a list of key words from the notes they took.	Share a Note: Students meet in small groups and share their notes with a partner. They discuss why they selected specific points.
Important to Me Students work in a small group at a table. In the center of the table is a chart where students can enter key phrases. After each student enters a phrase, the groups has a discussion about the key phrases.	Watch, Look, Listen: Students work in small groups and share their information with the other members of the group. Only one person speaks, and the other students are not allowed to talk except to ask a clarifying question. After everyone has had a turn, students can engage in conversation with their teammates.	Stations: Students write a critical point on an index card and leave it on a desk in one corner of the room. The class is divided into four groups and each group starts at a specific corner. After a group reads the notes at one corner of the room, they move to the next corner. Eventually they will circulate through the four corners.	My Summary: Students write a summary of what they learned and create a one-page note for the rest of the class.

The next chapter will look at the role of reflection in the instructional process and for self-regulation.

Please use the Student Interview rubric in the appendix to assess student learning.

REFERENCES

Duncan, C. A., and Clemons, J. M. (2012). Closure: It's more than just lining up. *Strategies*, 25(5), 30–32. Retrieved June 24, 2012, from http://www.ingentaconnect.com/content/aahperd/strat/2012/00000025/0000005/art0007.

Fisher, Douglas, and Frey, Nancy. (2004). *Improving Adolescent Literacy: Strategies at Work*. Upper Saddle River, NJ: Pearson Education.

Gardner, Howard. (2007). *Five Minds for the Future*. Boston, MA: Harvard Business School Press.

Marzano, R. L., Pinkering, D. J., and Pollock, J. E. (2001). *Classroom Instruction That Works: Re-*

search-Based Strategies for Increasing Student Achievement. Alexandria, VA: Association for Supervision and Curriculum Development.

Marzano, R. J. (2007). *Instructional Practices That Work*. Alexandria, VA: Association for Supervision and Curriculum Development.

Pastore, R. (2003). Dale's Cone of Experiences. Retrieved June 24, 2012, from http://teacherworld.com/potdale.html.

Phillips, L. (1987). Closure: The fine art of making learning stick. *Instructor*, *97*(3), 36–38. Retrieved June 24, 2012, from http://www.eric.ed.gov.

Restak, Richard. (2006). *The Naked Brain*. New York: Harmony Books.

Wolf, P., and Supon, V. (1994). Winning through student participation in lesson closure. [S. l.] Distributed by ERIC Clearinghouse. Retrieved June 24, 2012, from http://eric.ed.gov.

4

Lesson Design

Reflection

What is the value of reflection? How is reflection used in lesson design? Sample reflective questions are:

1. Was the Student Learning Target (SLT) objective met? If it was, how do I know students learned what was intended?
2. Were the students productively engaged? How do I know?
3. Based on formative assessments, did I need to alter my instructional plan? Why? What will I plan differently for the lesson next time I teach it?
4. What additional assistance, support, and/or resources would have further enhanced this lesson? How will they be incorporated into the lesson the next time I teach this lesson?
5. As I reflect upon the lesson, what would I do differently? Why?

Teachers can preplan their lessons by asking:

1. What do I expect the students to learn?
2. How will I know they are learning?
3. What questions will I build into the lesson to enhance student metacognition and rigor?
4. What activities will I plan so as to tier the lesson to differentiate student learning?
5. How will I close the lesson?

Table 4.1. Reflection Activity

How do I use reflection in my lesson planning?
What strategy seems to work best for reflection? Do I pause throughout the lesson or will I wait until after the lesson?
Do I meet with teachers during Common Planning Time (CPT), Professional Learning Communities (PLC), or grade-level meeting to reflect on lesson taught? How do I feel it worked or what would I change?
Do I work with teachers on Lesson Study whereby we bring a common lesson to a meeting and discuss what went well and what needs to improve? What did I learn and what will I do differently next time?

Why do I feel reflection is helpful?

Next steps/future action

WHAT IS REFLECTION AND HOW DOES IT RELATE TO TEACHERS AND STUDENTS IN THE CLASSROOM?

What comes to your educated mind when you hear the word reflection?

If you are like most people, you think of a mirror and how you observe yourself at that moment. When you use this looking glass, you either decide that everything is just fine, or you might decide to make changes to yourself. You will use your reflection to give serious thought and consideration to the matter of your looks. In education, we know the word reflection in a very similar way.

> Self-reflection allows a professional to think about where they are at that particular moment in their career and assess their practice. The teacher who is complacent and content should reconsider how they can improve their craft. As a teacher who has been through more than seven years of teaching English at primary and lower secondary levels, I have found myself in a position of a certain stagnation. At that phase, I started to ask myself more often; what [kind of] a teacher am I? [*sic*] To answer the question, I tried to look at my teaching from three different points of view (*Teacher Self-Reflection: Diploma Thesis*).

TEACHER REFLECTION: THE WHY

This introspection or reflection is defined as the self-observation and reporting of conscious inner thoughts, desires, and sensations. It is a conscious mental and usually purposive process relying on thinking, reasoning, and examining one's own thoughts, feelings, and actions. In education, this process is conducted to increase a student's academic output. When a teacher reflects upon her lesson, she is evaluating what went well or what can change for overall student improvement. Reflection, when used with the proper "self" questioning techniques and personal insight, ensures that the teacher will delve into the lesson from another perspective. When the teacher steps outside the box and reflects upon her accomplishments, she has not only grown professionally but personally as well. This teacher is making professional and personal connections with her students, which builds a successful foundation for everyone.

In order for educators to continually improve in the profession, it is necessary that they reflect upon their own teaching practice and ask deeper questions of what can be done differently, what worked and what did not work and what can be done to improve. It is this type of teacher reflection that is essential because it leads to consistent and constant improvement.

Reflection is also framed into shaping the environment. In his book *Experience and Education*, Dewey wrote that the primary responsibility of educators is that they not only be aware of the general principle of the shaping of actual experiences for the learner, but they also recognize what surroundings are conducive for having future experiences that lead to growth. As Dewey implies, teachers should know how to utilize the surroundings, both physical and social, that exist, so as to promote student self-regulation and contribute to building up experiences that are worthwhile.

Charlotte Danielson (2011, 2013) has developed a rubric for teacher reflection and teacher coaching. Her rubric has four domains and Domain 4 is titled "Professional Responsibilities." There are six components that address the teacher's professional skills. The components are reflection on practice, maintaining accurate records, communicating with families, participating in professional community, growing and developing professionally, and showing professionalism. The skills of Domain 4A, "reflecting on teaching," contain the essential elements of accuracy. Teacher reflection involves making a thoughtful and accurate assessment of a lesson's effectiveness and the extent to which it achieved its instructional outcome. In order to be effective, teachers should cite specific examples from the lesson and determine the relative strengths of each. What worked and why? How do I know?

It is the highly competent teacher, who reflects and understands what is necessary in the lesson, that is rated as distinguished or highly effective, while the teacher who does not know whether a lesson was effective or has achieved its instructional outcome is rated as unsatisfactory or ineffective.

Teachers need to distinguish among the various stages of the lesson reflection-*on*-action, which is what the students were doing as a result of the teacher's directive. Teacher reflection-*in*-action, and what is done during instruction. Teacher reflection-*for*-action is the desired outcome to the teach direction and the student action. Both reflection-in-action and reflection-on-action are essentially reactive in nature, being distinguished primarily by *when* reflection takes place. Reflection-in-action refers to reflection in the midst of practice (teacher directive or student directive) and reflection-on-action refers to reflection that takes place during an event (what did the student do as a result of the teacher's directive?). Reflection-for-action, on the other hand, is the desired outcome of the reflection. Did anything change?

In order for a teacher to be reflective-in-action, the teacher needs to receive feedback from students during or after she teaches the lesson. The teacher should think through what is happening, and with the information she is receiving from the students, she can reshape the lesson without stopping. She will determine if what she is doing is effective and understood by her students in this on-the-spot process. Based on the information that is received, the teacher can monitor and adjust her lesson. The monitoring and adjusting of the lesson contributes to reflection-on-action. Consequently, the teacher will be checking student outcomes frequently throughout the lesson, and she will use her feedback to **reflect** on whether she should reteach the concept or continue on with her lesson. Based on the reflection-in-action, the teacher will monitor and adjust the lesson accordingly. Reflection is an important component in the professional life of all teachers.

Table 4.2. Reflective Action Template

Reflection-on-action (What the students were doing as a result of the teacher's directive) 1. The teacher is monitoring and adjusting the lesson. 2. Adjustments are made based on the date. Comments:
Teacher reflection-in-action (What was done during instruction) 1. The teacher receives feedback from students during or after she teaches the lesson. 2. The teacher will monitor and/or adjust the lesson based on the feedback. Comments:
Teacher reflection-for-action (The desired outcome to the teacher direction.) 1. Did I get the desired student action? 2. As I reflect, should I re-teach the concept or continue on with the lesson? Comments:

Teacher Reflection

A short scenario may help you better understand this point. Consider the teacher that has just completed a lesson, or may be midway through a lesson with students. She finds that early on the lesson was going well, but then she begins to see her students yawning, chatting, and not as focused as she would expect. She stops ever so briefly, so as not to change the pace of her lesson, and does a quick personal evaluation of her teaching methods and then continues to complete the lesson. The students are unaware of her moment of pause or moment of reflection. The teacher may ask herself after the lesson:

Y/N	Do I need to change what I am doing as students are sending signals that they are bored? If no, what will I do next time?	
	What could I have done differently before I hit that bump in the lesson? *Reflection:*	
	What behavior would I want to see after I stop going forward? *I expect to see:*	
	What was the reaction of the students once I stopped the lesson? *Student reactions:*	
	Were there immediate changes within the classroom?	
	Did I miss an opportunity to *discipline* those "disruptive" students? If I did, what will I do next time if a similar situation occurs?	
	As I reflect, was the problem with the students or was this about the instructional delivery methodology?	
	Overall reflection:	

Our conclusion to this scenario may be that there was **no change** in the classroom atmosphere, yet the teacher continued with her lesson. We could also say that the no **immediate change** in the classroom was a result of her reflection and decision to continue her lesson. No matter what the answer to this scenario may be, the answer to all of the questions noted above is that this teacher should use **reflection** during her lesson. In addition, we strongly suggest that this teacher take more time after the lesson to reflect upon her own teaching. This teacher needs to examine what she actually did during the lesson, how and what she taught, and then come to a decision about what needs to be changed in order to better prepare the lesson for the next time she teaches it

Table 4.4. Teacher Reflection Questions

Was the lesson effective? Y/N What behavior did I see to support my conclusion?
How often did I monitor and adjust my instruction to ensure that students are learning?
What will I do if the lesson is not working?
Do I have alternative questions to ask the class to refocus their attention
Do I have a variety of activities planned for tiered lessons?
How will I address discipline problems? Will I use verbal and nonverbal strategies?

STUDENT REFLECTIONS

Why is reflective thinking important?

Modern society is becoming more complex, information is becoming available and changing more rapidly prompting users to constantly rethink, switch directions and change problem-solving strategies. Thus, it is increasingly important to prompt reflective thinking during learning to help learners develop strategies to apply new knowledge to the complex situation in their day to day activities. Reflective thinking helps learner develop higher order thinking skills by prompting learners to relate new knowledge to prior understanding, think in both abstract and conceptual terms, apply specific strategies in novel tasks, and understand their own thinking and learning strategies www.hawaii.edu/intlrel/pols382/Reflective%20Thinking%20-%20UH/reflection.html#bilbliography)

I agree with the quote because	I disagree because	Not sure because

Teachers, who model open-ended questioning techniques, stimulate student reflection, and deliberately generate the student's need to know more are providing strategies for students to use to become reflective and self-regulated learners. The use of open-ended questions helps begin the process of introspection and metacognition. The process of self-monitoring begins with student action, so it is important for the teacher to begin probing the student toward self-reflection in this way;

- ✓ Is the result you achieved what you had expected to achieve? Why?
- ✓ I am satisfied with the outcome because:
- ✓ If the outcome was not what you expected, what will you do differently?
- ✓ Will there be other resources or aides you can use to gain the desired result?
- ✓ Did you monitor your progress along the way or wait until the end? Was that an effective strategy?

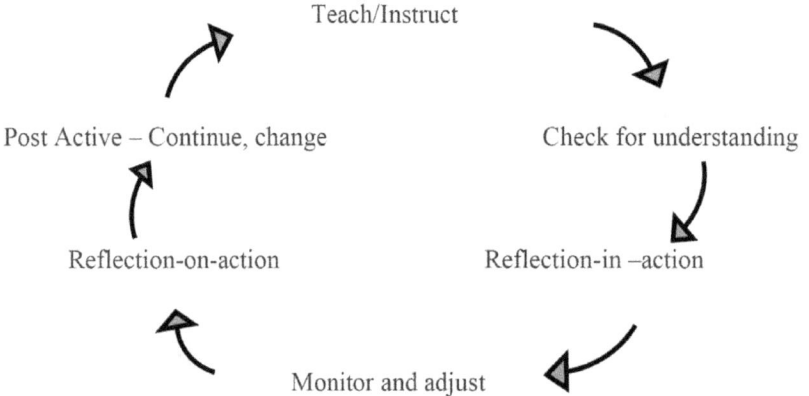

My flow chart looks like:

Teacher Reflection Flow Chart

HELPFUL QUESTIONS WHEN REFLECTING UPON A LESSON

- Were all students engaged in learning?

- Were less that 50 percent of the students engaged? Were the other students not engaged?

- What will I do to promote more student engagement?

- What evidence do I have that students understood what I hoped would come from the lesson?

- Did I do frequent checks for understanding?

- How did I monitor the lesson?

- Did I have activities available if I had to adjust the lesson?

- Did my anticipatory set begin as I anticipated?

- Did the lesson get off track? How?

- Were directions clear as students knew what to do and began their work immediately?

- Were materials accessible?

- As the activity progressed, how well did students remain focused?

- Was my grouping of students effective?

- Did students know how to monitor the quality of their work?

- Did students know how to get help or come to the teacher?

- How was the conclusion of the activity?

- What closure activity did I use and will I use it again?

Course of Action

_____

_____

_____

_____

_____

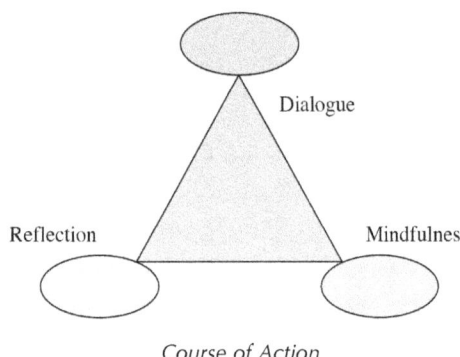

WHAT SHOULD YOU LOOK FOR IN YOUR TEACHING?

One of the hardest things to do as you begin to examine and think about your teaching practices is to figure out what is important and how to deliver that message. You may try to answer questions like the following:

✓ How do I determine what the students "know"?
✓ What level of questions do I ask? Is there a variety of questions being used?
✓ Do my questions scaffold the lesson?
✓ Do I use wait time effectively?
✓ Am I asking questions to find out what my students know or am I asking questions to move the lesson?
✓ Do my questions encourage students to think further about some idea: to explain, justify, or hypothesize?

- Am I using teacher wait time before and after I receive responses to questions to model the concept of wait time so students will use student-to-student wait time?
- Am I exploring alternative strategies posed by different students?
- Am I correcting unproductive thinking?
- Am I using various forms of communication: reading, writing, listening, and speaking?
- Am I modeling scientific thinking?
- What kind of questions are my students asking?
- Are my students talking to each other—disagreeing, challenging, and debating?
- Are my students willing to take risks?
- Are my students listening to each other?
- Are my students taking time to think about the problem, question, idea, or the like?
- Are my students able to explain their ideas clearly and precisely?
- Are my **students able to reflect** on the experience and identify what was hard or easy for them; what worked and what didn't; what they liked and what they didn't?

Aspect of the lesson	Focusing question	Planned Readiness	Outcome
Introduction: Readiness Set	Did the Readiness Set serve as a catalyst to begin the lesson?	Did the anticipatory set adequately activate prior knowledge?	Was prior knowledge activated? Did the level of questions posed indicate student activation of prior knowledge? Did students have "ah ha" moments?
Student Learning Target (Objective)	How did the Student Learning Target (SLT) or lesson objective get conveyed to the students during the lesson?	Were prompts and gestures used throughout the lesson to focus student attention on the SLT?	During independent practice, was the objective integrated into the lesson? Can students tell me what they were learning today? Can students state in their own words what they were learning?
Informational Stage	Did the students have the ability to apply the information that was presented or was the lesson teacher directed with little or no student activity?	How do I know that the students know and understand the information? What evidence will I be looking at to ensure student understanding?	How did the information derived from the use of formative assessments and checks for understanding impact the lesson?
Closure	How did the students react to the lesson? Did they demonstrate understanding of the lesson via a Demonstration of Learning (DOL) or from Evidence of Learning (EOL) activity?	Were overt or covert techniques used in the closure process? Do students prefer overt or covert closure activities?	Are different closure techniques planned for subsequent lessons? How will the information from the closure be used to plan subsequent lessons?
Summary	What will I keep?	What will I do differently for the next lesson?	What will change?

REFLECTION SHEET

I am upset because
_____

_____

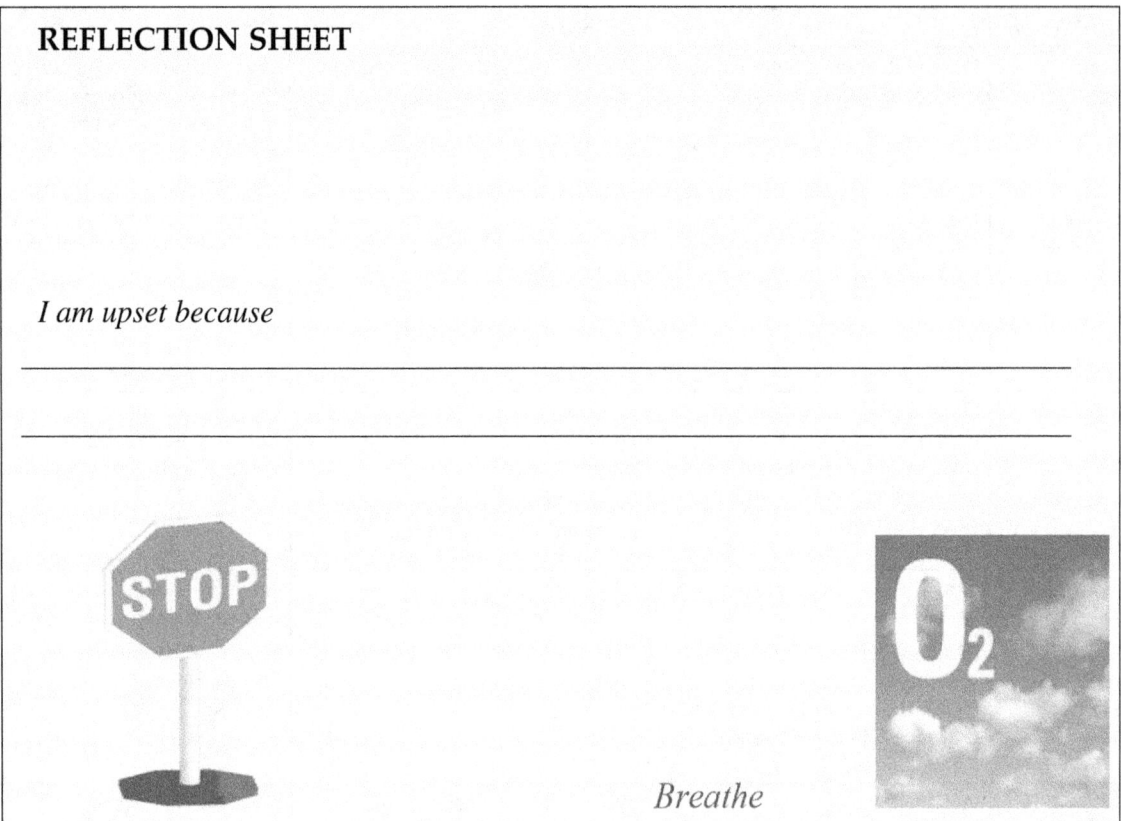

Breathe

Plan of Action

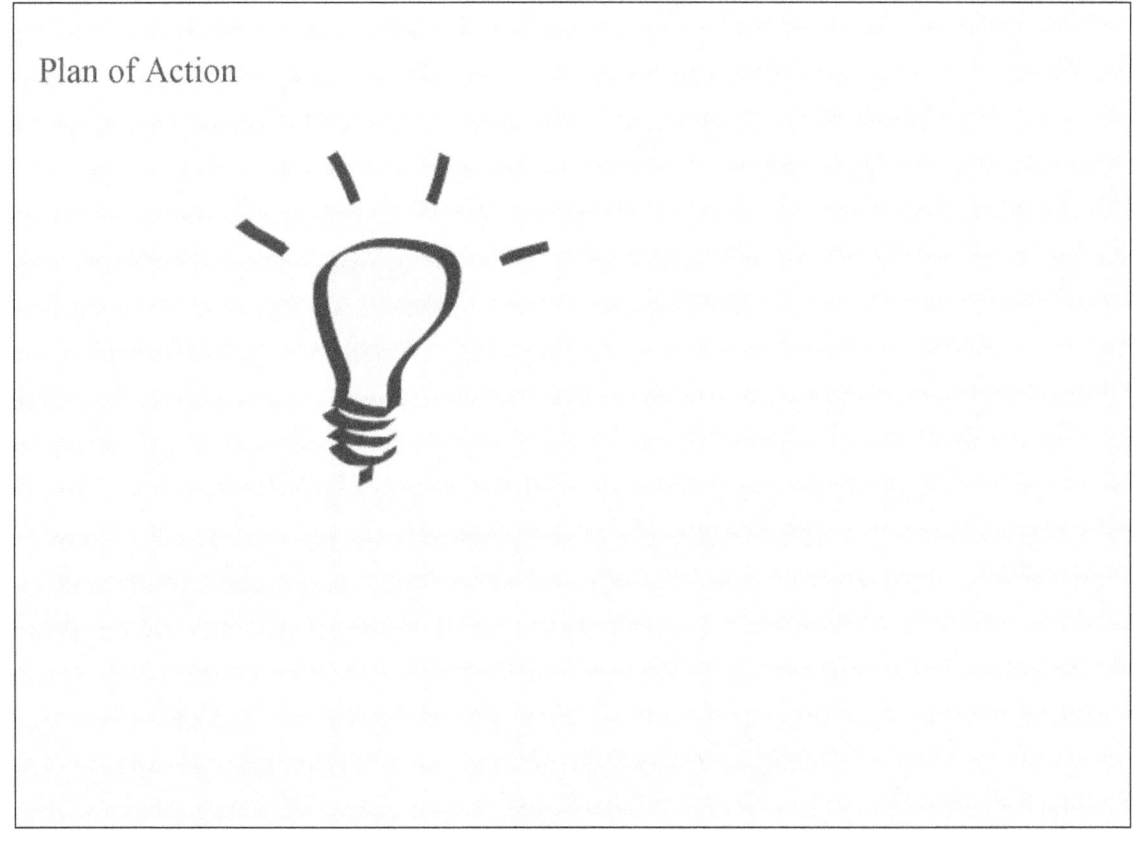

Reflect on the lesson you have developed and rate the degree to which the lesson meets the criteria below as either *Strong, Moderate,* or *Weak.*

Lesson Activities:	Suggested lesson reflection Strong, Moderate, or Weak	Rating: S?M?W?
1. Are they challenging and are higher-order thinking and problem-solving skills promoted? (Planning Stage) If not, why?	Were checks for understanding (CFU) done throughout the lesson? **S/M/W** If so, how did that information affect the lesson **S/M/W** *Comments*	
2. Student choice (Planning Stage)	Did students have the opportunity to select an activity for the lesson? **S/M/W** Did I monitor and regulate their learning throughout the independent lesson? **S/M/W** *Comments*	
3. Provide scaffolding for acquiring targeted knowledge/skills (Planning Stage/Instructional Stage)	What questions did I ask to scaffold the lesson? Were the questions effective in scaffolding the lesson? **S/M/W** *Comments*	
4. Did I plan my questions (Planning Stage)	Planned questions were effective? **S/M/W** *Comments*	
5. Integrate 21st century skills (Planning Stage)	Did I incorporate technology, digital citizenship, etc.? **S/M/W** *Comments*	
6. Provide opportunities for interdisciplinary connection and transfer of knowledge and skills (Planning Stage)	Did the cross-curricular activities I incorporated throughout help students make connections? **S/M/W** Did the students apply the learning across disciplines? **S/M/W** *Comments*	
7. Did I address different student learning styles?	Were my learning styles effective? **S/M/W**	
8. Was my lesson differentiated? **S/M/W** (Instructional Stage)	How do my students react to the tiered assignments? **S/M/W** *Comments*	

9. Is my differentiation based on student data? (Instructional Stage)	Were my formative assessments effective in helping me tier the lesson? **S/M/W** *Comments*	
10. Was the lesson student-centered with teacher acting as a facilitator and co-learner during the teaching and learning process? (Instructional Stage)	What was planned to determine if the students understood what was taught? Did it work? If not, what will be done differently? **S/M/W** Did I use a "gradual release" so the lesson was not teacher directed? **S/M/W** What will I do differently next time? Will I collect data early so I can make adjustments during the lesson? **S/M/W** *Comments*	
11. Did I provide means for students to demonstrate knowledge and skills and progress in meeting learning goals and objectives (DSL)	Was the DSL a good measure?	
12. Did I provide opportunities for student reflection and self-assessment (Closure)	Did the students use self-regulated strategies during the lesson? **S/M/W** *Comments*	
13. Provide data to inform and adjust instruction to better meet the varying needs of learners	What form of data collection did I use? What form of reporting did the students use? What was the outcome of the data? **S/M/W** (Instructional) *Comments*	
14. Closure planned?	What closure activity did I use and how successful was it compared to other closure activities I tried in the past? **S/M/W** (Closure) *Comments*	
Areas that were Strong	*Areas that were Moderate*	*Areas that were Weak*
	Next steps	*Next Steps*

REFERENCES

Christodoulou, Iva. (2010).Teacher self-reflection. Diploma thesis, Faculty of Education, Department of English Language and Literature, Masaryk University, Brno, Czech Republic. https://is.muni.cz/th/266245/pedf_m/DPIva_Christodoulou.pdf.

Creasap, Sally A., Peters, April L., and Uline, Cynthia L. (2005). The effects of guided reflection on educational leadership practice. *Journal of School Leadership*, *15*(4), 352–386. http://edweb.sdsu.edu/People/culine/880/Guided%20Reflection05.pdf.

Danielson, Charlotte. (2006). *Teacher Leadership that Strengthens Professional Practice*. Alexandria, VA: Association for Supervision and Curriculum Development.

Danielson, Charlotte. (2008). *The Handbook for Enhancing Professional Practice: Using the Framework for Teaching in Your School*. Alexandria, VA: Association for Supervision and Curriculum Development.

Danielson, Charlotte. (2011). *The 2011 Framework for Teacher Evaluation Instrument*. Princeton, NJ: The Danielson Group.

Danielson, Charlotte. (2013). *The 2013 Handbook for Teacher Evaluation Instrument* is available in PDF format from the Danielson Group website: www.danielsonfroiup.org.

Dewey, John. (1910). *How We Think*. Boston: D. C. Heath.

Dewey, John. (1916). *Democracy and Education*. New York: Free Press.

Dewey, John. (1933). *How We think: A Restatement of the Relation of Reflective Thinking to the Educative Process*. Chicago: Henry Regnery.

Dewey, John. (1938). *Experience and Education*. New York: Collier Books.

Jackson, Anthony. (2013). Japanese lesson study. *Global Learning. Education Week*, January 4, 2012.

Tomlinson, Carol Ann, and McTighe, Jay. (2006). *Integrating Differentiated Instruction and Understanding by Design: Connecting Content and Kids*. Alexandria, VA: Association for Supervision and Curriculum Development.

Yoshida, Makoto, and Fernandez, Clea. Overview of Lesson Study in Japan. *globaledresources.com*. rbs.org, Research for Better Schools, June 20, 2013.

5

Sample Lesson Plan

Putting It All Together

This chapter will provide a sample lesson and break down each component of the lesson. A special thank-you and acknowledgement to Christine Casale for providing the lesson plan. *Comments* are provided on how the lesson ties to the Learner's Brain Model.

LESSON PLANNING

Teacher's Name: Christine Casale
Lesson: Create an Advertisement
Unit Topic: Persuasive Writing
Grade level: 6th
Essential Questions: Why is persuasive writing important? How do we use persuasive writing in our own lives? How do we persuade others? How do persuasive messages influence us? What makes a good argument? Why is a writer's choice of words important? How do the rules of language affect communication? How do writers develop a well-written product?

Comment: *The essential question is consistent with the brain's processing of visual information in a holistic manner. In essence, the brain is looking for a pattern in which the visual—"visual thinking"—is connected to the end goal. Basically, the brain is looking to determine if there is a pattern in which a relationship to what is being taught is evident. We know this fact when we are all shown an optical illusion—we look to see a pattern but the illusion causes the visual impression to be compromised. It is the cognitive process of the new stimuli (the lesson) the student's current frame of reference that the brain is trying to sort out.* The Essential Question is the beginning of the pre-delivery (readiness stage) of the Learner's Brain Model.

STUDENT LEARNING TARGET (THE OBJECTIVE SHOULD BE STUDENT FRIENDLY)

I will be able to apply and evaluate persuasive strategies as well as use persuasive writing skills through oral discussion.

Comment: *Set objectives and provide feedback. This is important as this begins the process of self-regulation on the student's part. Most importantly, it is necessary to use prompts or gestures to refer back to the objectives and the essential question to focus student attention and "forward frame" the information for future use.*

Start and reinforce a lesson with questions and/ or advance organizers.

The Learner's Brain Model on lesson design addresses the issue of starting a lesson by using a Readiness Set. It helps to bridge to new information to motivate as well as focus the student.

STUDENT LEARNING TARGET (OBJECTIVE)

Comment: *An effective lesson will begin with the teacher ensuring that students are aware of the purpose and objectives of the lesson. Student Learning Targets (Objective) of the lesson should be clearly posted on the board or wall and will be reviewed with the class. The classroom teacher should communicate what the students should expect to learn during the lesson, why it is important, and what the students will be doing to achieve these objectives, otherwise the students are constantly searching for "meaning." If students understand the purpose and objectives of the lesson, it will help them assess themselves throughout the lesson to see if they are meeting the lesson objective so they are engaged in self-regulation. Do not set the instructional goals so specific and narrow as to lead the student to focus too narrowly on the goal and ignore other relevant information not specifically related to the goal. An effective objective ties in students' prior knowledge and connects to other parts of the students' curriculum and experiences. This will increase student engagement as the objective becomes more relevant and meaningful to the students.*

DEMONSTRATION OF STUDENT LEARNING (DSL)

Art Smart / Visual-Spatial student: I will create an advertisement and commercial using the writing process and receive at least a 3- on a 4-point rubric.

Verbal-Linguistic students: I will show the teacher I mastered the skill by completing a peer/self-assessment and evaluation form and sharing my results with the teacher in a teacher/student conference.

I will be able to review persuasive strategies and identifying strategies used in a passage and on Post-its, creating an advertisement and commercial using the writing process.

Interpersonal: I will complete peer/self-assessments and evaluation forms, sharing work, and participating in teacher/student conferences.

Comment: Lessons require daily Demonstrations of Student Learning (DSLs) by all students as it measures attainment of objectives. Additionally, the information obtained from the DSL will be useful for planning differentiated instruction. Keep in mind that the DSL is only one form of formative assessment, so using DSLs and checks for understanding, the teacher will be able to gain valuable information to monitor and adjust the instruction.

Standards to be Addressed

Comment: Use standards-based planning so students will know what the expectation level is that they are being held accountable to achieve. The standards will also allow feedback to be given to the student, based on established expectations and norms.

The use of standards will also help to bring focus to the teacher's planning and consistency to all teachers if all teachers across grade levels use them to plan. A problem would occur if some teachers were using one set of standards, for example, Common Core State Standards, and other teachers were using state standards different from the Common Core State Standards. Some standards may be covered at different grade levels so the curriculum would not be articulated.

WRITING

- CCSS.ELA-Literacy.W.6.1 Write arguments to support claims with clear reasons and relevant evidence.
  - CCSS.ELA-Literacy.W.6.1a Introduce claim(s) and organize the reasons and evidence clearly.
  - CCSS.ELA-Literacy.W.6.1b Support claim(s) with clear reasons and relevant evidence, using credible sources and demonstrating an understanding of the topic or text.
  - CCSS.ELA-Literacy.W.6.1c Use words, phrases, and clauses to clarify the relationships among claim(s) and reasons.

- CCSS.ELA-Literacy.W.6.1d Establish and maintain a formal style.
- CCSS.ELA-Literacy.W.6.1e Provide a concluding statement or section that follows from the argument presented.
- CCSS.ELA-Literacy.W.6.4 Produce clear and coherent writing in which the development, organization, and style are appropriate to task, purpose, and audience.
- CCSS.ELA-Literacy.W.6.5 With some guidance and support from peers and adults, develop and strengthen writing as needed by planning, revising, editing, rewriting, or trying a new approach.
- CCSS.ELA-Literacy.W.6.6 Use technology, including the Internet, to produce and publish writing as well as to interact and collaborate with others; demonstrate sufficient command of keyboarding skills to type a minimum of three pages in a single sitting.

COMPREHENSION AND COLLABORATION

- CCSS.ELA-Literacy.SL.6.1 Engage effectively in a range of collaborative discussions (one-on-one, in groups, and teacher-led) with diverse partners on grade 6 topics, texts, and issues, building on others' ideas and expressing their own clearly.
  - CCSS.ELA-Literacy.SL.6.1b Follow rules for collegial discussions, set specific goals and deadlines, and define individual roles as needed.
  - CCSS.ELA-Literacy.SL.6.1c Pose and respond to specific questions with elaboration and detail by making comments that contribute to the topic, text, or issue under discussion.
- CCSS.ELA-Literacy.SL.6.3 Delineate a speaker's argument and specific claims, distinguishing claims that are supported by reasons and evidence from claims that are not.

PRESENTATION OF KNOWLEDGE AND IDEAS

- CCSS.ELA-Literacy.SL.6.4 Present claims and findings, sequencing ideas logically and using pertinent descriptions, facts, and details to accentuate main ideas or themes; use appropriate eye contact, adequate volume, and clear pronunciation.
- CCSS.ELA-Literacy.SL.6.6 Adapt speech to a variety of contexts and tasks, demonstrating command of formal English when indicated or appropriate. (See grade 6 Language standards 1 and 3 here for specific expectations.)

CONVENTIONS OF STANDARD ENGLISH

- CCSS.ELA-Literacy.L.6.1 Demonstrate command of the conventions of standard English grammar and usage when writing or speaking.
- CCSS.ELA-Literacy.L.6.2 Demonstrate command of the conventions of standard English capitalization, punctuation, and spelling when writing.

KNOWLEDGE OF LANGUAGE

- CCSS.ELA-Literacy.L.6.3 Use knowledge of language and its conventions when writing, speaking, reading, or listening.
  - CCSS.ELA-Literacy.L.6.3a Vary sentence patterns for meaning, reader/listener interest, and style.
  - CCSS.ELA-Literacy.L.6.3b Maintain consistency in style and tone.

VOCABULARY ACQUISITION AND USE

- CCSS.ELA-Literacy.L.6.6 Acquire and use accurately grade-appropriate general academic and domain-specific words and phrases; gather vocabulary knowledge when considering a word or phrase important to comprehension or expression.

READINESS SET

The Learner's Brain Model uses a Readiness Set to get the student's interest at the onset of a lesson or at the beginning of a new lesson. After the Readiness Set, the teacher plans the lesson to "make sense" and have meaning for the student. This phase is Stage 1 of the Readiness Cycle.

The emphasis on setting the stage for learning fits precisely with the current research on the attentional mechanisms of the brain. Our brain immediately starts sifting and sorting through all the sensory input. At the same time, the brain searches through previously stored information and looks for relevant hooks for the new information. A Readiness Set increases the possibility that the brain will search through the right networks and attend to the information that is relevant for a particular topic or issue.

Examine the advertisement on the Smart Board. In your Do Now Journals, answer the following questions: What are they trying to sell? What persuasive strategies do they use? Are they successful? Students will share their responses with a partner, and the class will discuss the effectiveness of the advertisement as well as the strategies used.

Comment: The cognitive principle is that your "memory is not a product of what you remember, it is a product of what you think about" (Willingham, 2010, p. 43). The student needs to see the relationship of what they are learning so the material becomes relevant. To help achieve this concept, a Readiness Set is used to hook the student's interest, connect the student's prior knowledge and to tie both to the lesson so the lesson will make sense and have meaning.

The concept of Readiness Set is to focus student attention. The process is a way to help students organize and think about the content, see a direct link with what they previously studied, or help the student recall what they already know.

Instructional Input

This lesson will be part of a unit on persuasive writing. By this point, students will have been exposed to persuasive strategies such as testimonial and bandwagon.

Comment: The critical variable is that the teacher would have assessed their students to know where their students are and can plan appropriately. (Refer to chapter 2). Once the students are appropriately assessed, the teacher can tier the lesson based on student needs.

The purpose of the lesson is for students to not only develop their persuasive writing skills but apply these skills in a real-world context.

Comment: This is critical for authentic learning as students need to know what they are learning has application. If students do not see the application, the usual question is: "Why do we have to know this?" or the real killer question: "Will this be on the test?" If the teacher answers no, the student will fail to see the value of the information and may "shut down."

Students will review the persuasive strategies learned by discussing their review graphic organizer as well as identifying and evaluating strategies in sample advertisements around the room. After the review of the strategies, students will be responsible for creating their own advertisement and commercial in groups. The advertisement must use the persuasive strategies the class learned. It must include an illustration, slogan, and reasons to purchase the product or service. Students will also create a commercial where they must sell their product or service. They should create a jingle for the commercial. The advertisement and commercial must also include price comparisons and environmental implications of the product or service.

Comment: The use of creativity is important as students get to apply what they are learning in a new way.

If we teach for competency, we may not get performance. Students will know how to do a problem but lack the skill to apply it. If we teach for performance, where students have to show what they know, we automatically get competency. The Learner's Brain Model stresses metacognition via application so students develop competency and apply what they know.

VISUAL

A sample advertisement will be displayed on the Smart Board during the Do Now. Persuasive strategies with examples will be presented in a graphic organizer for easy reference. Sample advertisements will be posted around the room. Models, assignment rubric, and the assignment sheet will be shared with students and displayed on the Smart Board.

Comment: Using model and visual representations are stressed in math instruction and one of the new shifts for the Common Core. The Learner's Brain Model stresses establishing the physical environment, developing emotional security, mood, and climate as important for the classroom domain and to establish an environment conducive to learning. Establish a classroom environment so that safety, emotions, novelty, humor, music, choices, physical movement, hands-on activities can contribute to increased alertness and memory.

AUDITORY

Students will share their Do Now findings with a partner in a Think-Pair-Share activity. The class will discuss the Do Now findings as a large group as well. The teacher will review the persuasive strategies through oral discussion when referencing the graphic organizer. After reviewing the handout, students will be asked to share with a partner at least three strategies they think are most effective. The class will also review the sample advertisements together after students label them with Post-it notes. The teacher will review the models, rubrics, and assignment sheets, orally asking students questions and providing students with the opportunity to also ask questions.

Upon completion of the entire project, students will share with the class. As groups are presenting the advertisement and commercial, the rest of the class will complete an evaluation form noting the persuasive strategies used. As a large group, the class will discuss their findings and the effectiveness of the advertisements and commercials.

Research has also shown that while threats impede learning, positive emotional experiences, during which the brain produces certain chemicals or neurotransmitters, can promote learning.

Comment: Research has shown that the brain's limbic system, located just above the brain stem at the base of the brain, is responsible for our emotional responses. Neuroscientists have determined that new information that comes to the brain is processed first in the emotional center before being processed in the cognitive center, located in the frontal lobe of the cerebrum. With information processing short-circuited first to the emotional center, chronic stress may impair long-term memory and learning. The effects of stress on learning have significant implications for educators, hence why the Learner's Brain Model stresses establishing a safe emotional environment for students so they can participate in class discussion, debates, or critiques of their peers' work or presentation.

TACTILE

Students will respond to the Do Now by writing in their journals. To review persuasive strategies, students will be shown various sample advertisements. They must be able to write the persuasive strategy used in the sample advertisements on a Post-it note.

KINESTHETIC

Students will then have to place their Post-it note under the correct advertisement.

CONCRETE SEQUENTIAL

Rubric and assignment sheet will be provided to present tasks in an organized manner. Rubrics are used as checklists to self-regulate. Models and sample advertisements will be shown and can be referenced freely throughout the class. The teacher will conference with students to ensure expectations are clear. Students are making original products because they are creating an advertisement. They also are creating graphs and charts for the price comparisons. Creating the advertisement and commercial are hands-on activities to a practical problem that require realistic writing.

ABSTRACT SEQUENTIAL

Models and sample advertisements will be shown. Part of the assignment requires an illustration. Research of prices and environmental implications is also necessary. The project requires problem-solving skills and synthesis to convey one clear advertising goal based on reason. The element of argument is present because students are constructing persuasive advertisements to convince others to purchase their product or service. There is also individualized study because each group member has specific tasks to accomplish. Lecture is used when the project is introduced. Outlining and note taking will also be used in the brainstorming stage.

CONCRETE RANDOM

Students will be working in small groups. There is an aspect of problem solving and use of real-world experience in the lesson because they need to determine how to market their product. Students are creating an advertisement and commercial, which requires innovation and divergent thinking as well as a hands-on experience. Brainstorming and gathering information is needed before creating the final product.

Comment: Use real materials such as familiar, tangible objects to demonstrate concepts and make ideas more concrete. For example, when teaching about ice, water, steam, use real-life objects to learn the concepts.

Use chants and rhymes while learning as rhythmic patterns stick to the brain.

Movement and humor are also important. Dance, sign, play games, and laugh as these activities will use multiple sense and will increase memory.

ABSTRACT RANDOM

Students will be working in small groups on varying tasks with benchmarks for completion. Models of the project will be shared. Teacher feedback is provided to all students throughout the entire project. Illustration is part of the requirement for the advertisement and role playing is required in the commercial. There is also an element of music necessary in the commercial for the jingle. Creative writing is also needed for both the commercial and advertisement.

Modeling

The teacher will review the persuasive strategies presented on the graphic organizer. The teacher will then reference the sample advertisements around the room. Students must determine which strategies are used in the advertisements and if they are effective. The teacher will model how to determine the persuasive strategies used in the first advertisement. After students review the persuasive strategies, the teacher will review the rubric and assignment sheet for the advertisement and commercial with students, so expectations are clear. The class will be presented with several models and a rubric that can be referenced freely throughout the class. Students will have an opportunity to ask questions.

Comment: During this time, the instructor will share with the class a time they have received help from an unlikely source. The instructor will help the students understand that sometimes you may receive help without even realizing it. The instructor will help the students prepare for the lesson through this discussion by scaffolding into the story for the class.

Input (Activities)

Students will share with a partner three persuasive strategies that they find most effective. The teacher will then ask students to examine the sample advertisements around the room and on a Post-it note write the strategy they think is being used. Students will be asked to place their Post-it note under the advertisement.

After review of the first activity, students will be divided into randomly selected groups, where each student will be assigned specific tasks to complete. Each group will receive a card with a product or service like cereal or bakery. However, they are able to make the product or service their own by creating its own brand, including a name and identifying features. Students must complete brainstorming and rough drafts prior to completing the final project. Students will use a rubric throughout the project for self-assessment purposes. They will complete a group assessment rubric at the end of the lesson to ensure that all students are accountable for contributing to the group.

Comment: The more senses involved during learning, the more likely the brain will receive and process information. By using multiple senses to learn, children find it easier to match new information to their existing knowledge.

The brain performs many functions simultaneously. Learning is enhanced by a rich environment with a variety of stimuli.

Hands-on activities increase sensory input which helps learners attend better.

Present content in a variety of teaching strategies, such as physical activities, individual and group instruction, artistic and musical variations, to help orchestrate student experiences.

Guided Practice

The teacher will circulate and monitor progress when students are recording the strategy on the Post-it notes.

Comment: After the teacher feels comfortable with the progress of the lesson, keeping in mind the notion of primary-recency, there may be a point in the lesson for students to do independent practice. The teacher monitors the student's progress and ensures that the student has the knowledge and appropriate skill to do the activity independently. The research done by Marzano, Pickering, and Pollack revealed that mastering a skill requires focused practice and even suggests that it's not until students have practiced "upwards of about 24 times that they reach 80 percent competency" (Marzano et al., 2001, p. 67).

Once in groups for creating the advertisement and commercial, the teacher will monitor progress and circulate among groups to make sure that students are staying on task and answer any questions. Students must first brainstorm using a graphic organizer. As students complete brainstorming and rough drafts, they will be shown to the teacher before creating the final project. The teacher and student will discuss strengths and areas in need of improvement.

Check for Understanding

To ensure students understand the strategies before moving onto the group part of the project, the teacher will review the identified strategies students wrote on the Post-it notes and students will discuss the effectiveness. The teacher will also encourage students to ask questions after discussion of the project so expectations are clear.

Once in groups, the teacher will check brainstorming and rough drafts of each group prior to creating the final product. The teacher will chunk activities and give estimated completion times. Groups will provide the teacher with status updates of their projects. Students will share their graphic organizer with a partner and be encouraged to ask their group questions for clarification throughout the project. Students will use a rubric to self-assess and peer editing throughout the project to self-regulate and ensure they are on task. Once the project is completed, students will also present their projects, complete evaluation forms, and engage in large group discussion about the effectiveness of the advertisements/commercials.

Comment: During the activity, there will be frequent checks for understanding using a variety of strategies. The instructor will see if the children understand what was being said and if their answers are accurate by sharing their answers with the class. During this time, the students will be chosen randomly to help get all the students involved in the discussion and to make sure the children are participating. Participation is not optional. At this time the class will construct a KWL chart based upon the answer sheets. This chart will help to show what the class already knows, learned, and what they want to learn in this lesson. This chart will be held in the front of the class and will be added to as the information is learned or if there is anything new that the students may want to learn. This chart will be an ongoing process in this lesson

The teacher can also use other ways to check for understanding—visual, tactile, or kinesthetic.

MULTIPLE INTELLIGENCES

Linguistic

Students will use their persuasive writing skills to create the advertisement and commercial. Students must consider their target audience. They must brainstorm convincing reasons to purchase their product or service as well as what differentiates their product or service from competitors. They must also create a slogan. Specific persuasive strategies must be used.

Logical–Mathematical

The students must show the price of their product or service in comparison to other competitors, using graphs and charts in their advertisement and commercial. (Computers will be used to research price comparisons.)

Musical

Students will create a commercial to sell their product or service using persuasive strategies. As part of the commercial, students can add a jingle.

Bodily–Kinesthetic

Students will create a commercial to sell the product or service. They will have to physically act out the commercial. Students will need to move freely around the room to work with others and gather supplies for each task.

Spatial–Visual

Students will be asked to create an illustration as part of the advertisement. The picture should support the persuasive strategies used.

Interpersonal

Students will be working collaboratively in groups throughout the entire project. Students must be able to ask questions of their peers and share progress. Work must be divided; however, through collaboration, it must all communicate the same persuasive goal.

Intrapersonal

Each student within the group will have certain tasks to accomplish independently.

Naturalist

Students were encouraged to make their product/service environmentally friendly, so they must examine the environmental implications of their project. (Computers may be used to research environmental impact of product or service.)

LESSON PLAN

Teacher: Ms. Smith/ Gr. 2

Focus: Author's Purpose

Student Learning Target (Objective)

I will be able to identify the author's purpose and justify my reasoning.

Demonstration of Learning (DSL)

I will correctly identify three important element of the story and provide supporting evidence for my choices to justify my answers.

Read Aloud: "Schools around the World"

Cross-Content Connection: Social Studies

Standards: *RF2.3f, RF2.4c, SL 2.1a, L2.6,*

OPENING/ MINI-LESSON

Brief Vocabulary Review: Prior to beginning the lesson, five-minute review on key vocabulary. Re-teach strategies on decoding and word analysis for vocabulary words. These are words that are present in the story and will increase vocabulary development. For students who need additional support, handout of the definitions with pictures will be provided.

Diverse: things or people that are different from each other
Literacy: the ability to read and write
Resources: materials, money, and other things that can be used
Culture: a group's customs or traditions
Uniform: clothes that all of the people in a group wear so they are dressed alike
Proper: the way it is supposes to be; correct

Display pictures of schools and classrooms from different countries on the board. Open the discussion by triggering the students' memory.
Comment: This will get their attention and make it meaningful.
Ask the children to discuss some memories from their school experience. After a few selections, refer to the pictures of different schools. Allow students to note details in the picture by comparing and contrasting their lives and the pictures.
Comment: Brain research says the frontal lobe is processing information when students talk. Talking and walking promotes metacognition.
Comment: A Readiness Set in this lesson involves a think-pair-share activity that is extremely important because brain research has found that learning is emotional and that permanent learning almost always has an emotional component. Memory and learning are closely tied to emotions. Having the students interact with one another works best because it gets the students interested and engaged in their own learning. In addition, the brain remembers information more readily

when it is meaningful and can be linked to prior knowledge or experience.

On the gathering area, display a KWL graphic organizer on a chart. Discuss with the children that we are going to read a book about schools around the world. Filling in the chart together, ask students questions for each section of the KWL chart. What do you know? What do you want to know? And afterwards, what have you learned? Each section will be color coded for easy reference.

Comment: Brain research explains using color increases learning.

Inform the students that the essential question is related to the author's purpose. "What is the purpose of the selection?" "Why did the author write this story?" Call on two students to make a prediction about the story. (Begin reading the story.)

Comment: Throughout the story, stop and ask questions about the literature. This will give the students the opportunity to engage in critical thinking: hypothesize, predict, visualize, evaluate, and draw conclusions. As discussed in the text, prediction has value in promoting retention. Prediction is also a great tool for increasing comprehension. After the story, we will summarize and discuss important details from the story.

Comment: Address all levels of Revised Bloom's taxonomy—literal, inferential, and creative levels. It is suggested that teachers continue to effectively engage students in meaningful ways and differentiate instruction based on students' readiness and academic needs. Essential questions written in plan books and posted in classrooms will assist teachers in developing more rigorous questioning types. Thoughtful lesson planning that targets higher-order thinking skills enables students to "get the big picture" and transfer learned knowledge to new and different situations.

In order for students to be actively engaged in learning, the students need to be mentally involved in understanding the lesson content and are participating and contributing to the instructional lesson. *The teacher needs to be asking cognitively challenging questions that will ensure that the students are thinking. Questions should have more than one answer and should not be simple "yes" or "no" questions. Research indicates that questions that require students to use higher-level thinking skills produce more metacognition than questions that require students to recall or recognize information. It is important to allow "wait" time after posing a question as this will allow a greater depth of student responses. In addition, all classroom activities and assignments should require students to think broadly and deeply, problem solve, and engage in critical thinking.*

WORK PERIOD

Distribute a number to each child from one to four. There will be four traveling stations in the classroom. The number will determine the students' placement. At each station, there will be a question related to the story and four minutes for each member to answer. Students will discuss opinions and experiences regarding the lesson. After four minutes, the timer will go off and each group will move to the next station. Once the groups are at their starting point, students will return to their seats for independent work. Students will complete a Venn diagram comparing and contrasting our school and the schools in the story.

Comment: Hands-on activities increase sensory input which helps learners attend better. It is important for the teacher to monitor student progress when they are working in small groups or student talk becomes unproductive or a "huddle" (students gather together and talk).

CENTERS

Comment: The brain is always seeking the big picture—the pattern of thought that is created by repeated use of familiar neural pathways.

Listening Center

Listen to "Schools around the World." Students can listen to the same story on tape. Those students having difficulty with comprehension or low-leveled readers can use the audio and picture book for assistance.

Writing Center

Students will write five facts about our school. They will also draw a picture to go with their sentences.

Technology Center

Teacher will provide appropriate websites for students to use.

Free-Time Center (Sensory Enrichment)

Students will have a variety of materials and resources to explore and stimulate conversations with each other. This center allows for discovery and explanation from areas such as foods, geography, family, community, senses, etc.

Guided Reading (Group 3)

Focus: Author's Purpose. Read the story "What We Do in Schools." Use this story to connect it to the read-aloud from the opening lesson. This is also an opportunity for increased personal connections.

CLOSING MEETING

The students will reconvene in the gathering area. We will restate our objective and discuss the story again. Some students will be called upon to share their Venn diagram. Teacher will also call upon one person from each center to discuss what they did and how it connected to today's lesson. The students will complete our KWL chart. Teacher will also ask students questions regarding the story to informally check for understanding.

Comment: The nature of classroom talk is complicated and too little understood. While there is evidence that more "thoughtful" classroom talk leads to improved reading comprehension (Fall, et al., 2000; Johnston et al., 2001; Nystrand, 1997), *especially in high-poverty schools* (Knapp, 1995), *we still have few interventions available that focus on helping teachers develop the instructional expertise to create such classrooms and few of the packaged programs offer teachers any support along this line. True conversation cannot be scripted or packaged. The classroom talk observed should be highly personalized and focused on a targeted reply to student responses. Teacher expertise is the key, not a scripted, teacher-proof, instructional product.*

Below is an example of how to incorporate the DI rubric for *Grade 2 Everyday Math Lesson Data Day* by Mrs. Dorothy Lusk. Mrs. Lusk is the general education teacher in the grade two inclusion classroom at William J. McGinn Elementary School, Scotch Plains, New Jersey. She has been teaching for 14 years in the primary classroom including kindergarten, first, and second grade. Mrs. Lusk incorporates her special-education background into the regular education classroom in order to meet the needs of the varied learners, from students who receive support and pull-out services to very bright and highly motivated students. Differentiation occurs both through varying academic difficulty and varying modalities of learning in order to provide many ways for students to access instruction at a level that is both developmentally appropriate and engaging.

DIFFERENTIATED INSTRUCTION

The following lesson is from Grade 2: *Everyday Math*. In the past Mrs. Lusk taught the lesson using the procedures from steps 1 to 8; step 9 has been created and added to this lesson to follow Differentiated Instruction Activities. Additionally, she adapted the Differentiated Instruction Chart, page 2, copyrighted by Dr. Mario Barbiere, to be used as a tool to check on the effectiveness of this specific lesson and its components. The chart could be used to check any lesson for Differentiated Instruction. Each of the lessons' tasks and activities are aligned according to the standards of highly effective with student engagement in the areas of content, process, product, interest, and readiness "look fors."

Comment: The rubrics can be used for preplanning a lesson, during a lesson, or reflection after a lesson.

Math: Lesson 6.3 Data Day NEED CIRCULARS

CCCS: 2.MD.5, 2.MD.10

Vocabulary: basic food groups, Food Guide Pyramid, data table, bar graph

OBJECTIVES

1. I will demonstrate the ability to collect, sort, tally and graph data.
2. I will demonstrate the ability to locate and identify food items in the food groups using a grocery store circular as a connection to real life.
3. I will be introduced to the concept of science and nutrition as it is connected to everyday math and real life.
4. I will demonstrate an understanding of the reality of limited spending within a budget.
5. I will demonstrate the ability to create a daily menu to reflect an understanding of a balanced diet and without and within budgetary restrictions.

PROCEDURES

1. The teacher will display a model of the old version of the 5 Basic Food Groups on the ELMO as the Guidelines for Second Graders: Lead a discussion regarding how the food groups work and what each part means.

    Comment: The more senses involved during learning, the more likely the brain will receive and process information. By using multiple senses to learn, children find it easier to match new information to their existing knowledge.

2. The teacher will guide the students in a shared reading activity in which each student views his/her own math journal page depicting the new U.S. Dept. of Agriculture model of Food Groups. Each group will work together on the task: Compare the two models and create a list of what you notice to share with the class: You should notice both similarities and differences. Allow the students to notice that the pyramid is divided into six parts because the U.S. Dept. of Agriculture divided up the fruits/vegetables and added a category for fats/sweets (TE 391).

    Comment: Brain research shows that lifelong learning best occurs when students are able to apply content, skills, and processes to tasks that require them to engage in higher-order thinking and problem-solving skills.

    Using knowledge meaningfully requires students to extend thinking by examining concepts in deeper, analytical ways, thus requiring the brain to use multiple and complex systems of retrieval and integration. Modules from one part of the brain connect to other modules when we perform complex tasks. Problem-solving activities that include cognitive components such as memory, language, emotion, and active learning engages the motor cortex.

    Limit the number of new concepts taught per day. For example, when teaching first graders about food groups, begin with only one food group at a time.

Summarizing and note taking reduces the amount of information the learner needs to get into long-term storage. Each is a form of a chunking strategy.

Children are better able to focus on important information when they receive less, rather than more, information.

When you reduce the amount of information to be learned, there is a better chance for it to be stored in the long-term storage.

3. The teacher will tell the class that today as part of our study of Food Groups they will be choosing various activities to learn about the Food Groups and how they fit in everyday life.

    Comment: Classroom rituals and specific opening and closing routines provide beginning and endings of class segments and also add an emotional component and help to establish a safe environment for students as everyone knows classroom expectations. It also helps to establish classroom management procedures.

4. The teacher will display grocery store circulars and pose the question: Have you ever seen one of these? What is it? What could we use it for? How does it help a consumer?

    Comment: The Readiness Set also helps to establish a readiness for what will be coming and to establish a safe emotional environment.

The Readiness Set in this lesson involves a think-pair-share activity that is extremely important because brain research has found that learning is emotional and that permanent learning almost always has an emotional component. Memory and learning are closely tied to emotions. Having the students interact with one another works best because it gets the students interested and engaged in their own learning. In addition, the brain remembers information more readily when it is meaningful and can be linked to prior knowledge or experience.

5. The teacher will allow the students to peruse the circulars briefly. She will have the students discuss what they notice about the circulars with their table groups and quickly share out their observations, including: format, location of items by category, pictures, prices and varieties of product (name brands / store brands). She will tell the students they will be using the circulars at some of the Choice Board activities. The task is to engage the students emotionally in the lesson.

    Comment: Emotions drive attention, attention drives learning and memory. Things become real to the brain when we feel them emotionally. Emotions affect memory and brain functions. Jensen (2005) notes that when a person feels content, the brain releases endorphins that enhance memory skills.

6. Before separating the group, the teacher will ask every student to write down their favorite meal (e.g., pizza, salad, and Diet Coke).

7. Tell the students they will be working with their partner to list the ingredients that are used to make up their favorite meal (dough: bread/grains, mozzarella cheese: dairy, tomato sauce: vegetables, salad: vegetables, dressing: fats/oils, Diet Coke: no food value). Once this is done, these will be collected for use in one of the Choice Board activities.

8. The students will be divided into groups/partners with various tasks from the Choice Board assigned to differentiate this lesson. Hands-on manipulation increases the chance by 75 percent that new information will be stored in long-term memory (Hannaford, 1995, Sousa, 2006. Hands-on activities increase sensory input which helps learners attend better.

Table 5.1.

	Anchor Activities	Choice Board (#9)
Whole Class	Introduction (#1) Display and Distribute Circulars (#5)	• Create a life-size Food Pyramid on class bulletin board; students take turns cutting items out of their circulars and placing them in the correct category of the Food Pyramid.
Individual	Shared Reading Food Pyramid (#2) Favorite Meal (#7)	• Use the circulars to locate prices for favorite food in order to make the meal. • Write journals: Do you think making healthy food choices is important? Explain why or why not.
Partner	Ingredients of Favorite Meal (#8)	• Create graphs based on tally chart of favorite food ingredients for Food Pyramid. Graph choices • **Low**—picture or bar graph with assistance to determine set up of graph. • **Middle**—bar graph agreed upon set up by the partners with mode and range identified. • **High**—pie graph with percentages/fractions identified and marked. • Use the menu costs to determine change from a given dollar amount (possible amounts: $20.00, $50.00, $100.00).
Small Group	Compare Food Pyramids (#3) Peruse Circulars / Compare Circulars (#6)	• Tally chart of Favorite Food Ingredients for Food Pyramid categories. • Set up menu for the day with balanced food choices. • Use the menu and circulars to estimate a realistic cost of the menu. • Complete a balanced menu within a budget. • Analyze the cost of each category of the pyramid; Is one category more expensive than another?

Table 5.2. Adapted from Differentiated Instruction Table.

Dispositions- "Look fors"	*Highly Effective Student Engagement*	*Highly Effective Considerations or Tasks*	*Specific Math Lesson Objectives/ Procedures/Activities* *Highly Effective*
Content "Look fors" Standards based, inter- disciplinary, rigorous, student centered, authentic	<ul><li>Whole group lesson leads to: individual, partner, and small group activities.</li><li>Teacher-directed and student-selected activities.</li><li>*The teacher will guide the students in a shared reading activity in which each student views his/ her own math journal page depicting the new U.S. Dept. of Agriculture model of Food Groups*</li></ul>	<ul><li>Interdisciplinary lesson with high level of application</li><li>Problem-based learning demonstrates deeper understanding. *Each group will work together on the task: Compare the two models and create a list of what you notice to share with the class; you should notice both similarities and differences. Allow the students to notice that the pyramid is divided into six parts because the U.S. Dept. of Agriculture divided up the fruits/ vegetables and added a category for fats/sweets (TE 391)*</li><li>Analysis promotes understanding</li></ul>	<ul><li>Interdisciplinary Lesson: Math/ Science/Social Skills/Health</li><li>Whole Group: (see above chart)</li><li>Individual: (see above chart)</li><li>Partner: (see above chart)</li><li>Small Group: (see above chart)</li><li>Teacher Directed: Introduction to Lesson - Food tables</li><li>Student Selected: Choice Boxes</li><li>Problem-Based Learning Activity:</li><li>Food Choices, Costs, Graphing</li></ul> *The grouping of students into high, middle, and low will allow for student interest, student readiness, and student product to be factored into the lesson for differentiation.*
Process "Look fors" Structured, dynamic, monitored, and adjusted based on feedback; promotes Self- Regulated Learning (SRL)	<ul><li>Students move at own pace and self-manage their time</li><li>*Student selects activities in addition to anchor activity*</li><li>*Flexible grouping is used to group students*</li><li>*Students use multiple intelligences*</li></ul>	<ul><li>Centers set up with materials needed</li><li>Students work with partner or small group and manage their time to complete the activity</li><li>Choice Board is posted to chose activity; mandatory activity is in place for all to manage</li></ul>	Time schedule is posted to complete each activity and each student has his/ her own folder to manage materials when time is called *Anchor Activity:* Center and Choice Boards to determine each student-selected activity *Multiple Intelligences:* Visual/ Spatial: use of circulars, food pyramids, graphs, and tally charts Body/Kinesthetic: awareness of proper diet, moving around to various centers Logical/Mathematical: calculating the cost of food items and determining how to fit within a given budget Verbal/Linguistic: use of written and oral language to complete various charts and graphs and explain results or findings Intrapersonal: metacognition, thinking about what is best for healthy diets and determining which food group a choice belongs to and identifying own food choices - ability to balance healthy and unhealthy Interpersonal: Working with a partner or small group cooperatively

Product "Look fors" Summative, diverse, MI used, shows what students know, understand, or do	• Real-world application • *Use MI to create product based on student ability* • Information is analyzed, interpreted, and created	• Activities demonstrate what each student knows and understands or can do independently and in a small group or partnership	• Using circulars to make food menu choices for a balanced meal • Using circulars to estimate costs and compute real costs within a budget • *Multiple Intelligences: student-selected choices encompass various learning styles as outlined in above chart* • Food choices are analyzed for nutritional balance and cost • Menus are created according to given criteria
Interest "Look fors" Student-involvement activities, student connections, self- regulation	• Specific references to students' interests are highlighted throughout the activities • *Real-world student connection is made* • Students self-regulate their choices	• *Tasks involve real-world procedures and expectations for daily living* • Students identify their own choices and complete the assignments based on personal choice not on one-size-fits-all choice	Students choose foods according to own likes and preferences • *Real-world connections* • *Healthy diets lead to long lives* • *Living within a budget* • *Favorite foods are used as a hook to generate interest*
Readiness "Look fors" Student skill levels, grouping, assessments to determine levels	• Pre-assessments are made to determine grouping • *Teacher assistance/ resources are available for students with special needs in order to have same level of choice as typical peers* • *Writing journals: Do you think making healthy food choices is important? Explain why or why not is an example of promotion of self- regulation. The teacher will review student journals to determine what feedback can be given to promote self-regulation.*	• Each specific task has more than one level of difficulty, depending on the task • *Final products based on MI.* • *Using MI is one way to provide a way of understanding intelligence, which teachers can use as a guide for developing classroom activities that address multiple ways of learning and knowing. Teaching strategies informed by MI theory transfers control from teacher to learners by giving students choices in the ways they will learn and demonstrate their learning.*	Food Pyramid on ELMO compared/ contrasted with New Guidelines Pyramid • Grouping for graphing based on previous graphing activities outside of this activity • Making change amount is also based on previous estimating and making change activities outside of this activity • In-class support teacher is available to assist with or modify activities as needed in addition to predetermined groupings • Some activities are leveled within the task • Final Products based on MI

MRS. LUSK REFLECTION

After my own analysis of how to differentiate the lesson, I realize how much more student directed the learning becomes with a relatively small amount of teacher-directed instruction to enable the students to complete many tasks that include a real-world application and meaning.

Regardless of what evaluation model a district uses, New Jersey teachers are being evaluated based on the rigor of the lesson, the quality of questioning involved, the real-world application of the student activities, the actual knowing and understanding of the product, the ability of the students to self-regulate their learning in a meaningful manner, and the assessment of the learning in order to generate future lessons and ways to best instruct the students. Interdisciplinary instruction is also becoming the only way to fit the increasing demands of a vast and demanding curriculum.

As for our students, differentiated instruction enables all students to learn to their highest potential by virtue of the use of multiple intelligences and a variety of tasks designed to meet all learners' needs not a one-size-fits-all model. Differentiated Instruction takes practice and requires a commitment, however, productive learning leads to application far beyond simply that lesson and the application is what truly demonstrates understanding and the acquisition of useful knowledge.

REFERENCES

Anderson, L.W., Krathwohl, D.R., Airasian, P.W., Cruikshank, K.A., Mayer, R.E., Pintrich, P.R., Raths, J., and Wittrock, M.C. (2001). *A Taxonomy for Learning, Teaching, and Assessing: A revision of Bloom's Taxonomy of Educational Objectives*. New York: Pearson, Allyn & Bacon.

Bloom, B. S. (1956). *Taxonomy of Educational Objectives: The Classification of Educational Goals Handbook I: Cognitive Domain*. New York: David McKay Company.

Caine, R. N., and Caine, G. (1990, October). Understanding a brain-based approach to learning and teaching. *Educational Leadership*, 48(2).

Caine, R. N., and Caine, G. (1990). Understanding a brain-based approach to learning and teaching. *Educational Leadership 48* (2).

Dalton, J., and Smith, D. (1986). Extending Children's Special Abilities–Strategies for Primary Classrooms, pp. 36–37; http://www.teachers.ash.org.au/researchskills/dalton.htm

Danielson, Charlotte. (2007). *Enhancing Professional Practice: A Framework for Teaching* (2nd ed.). Alexandria, VA: Association for Supervision and Curriculum Development.

Detchen, J. French, Accent on Teaching,. New York: Harper & Bros., 1954.

Elder, Janet. Findings about Brain Research and Brain-Friendly Instructional Strategies. www.readingprof.com

Elder, Janet. Findings about Brain Research and Brain-Friendly Instructional Strategies. www.readingprof.com.

Hannaford, C. (1995). *Smart Moves: Why Learning is Not All in Your Head*. Arlington, VA: Great Ocean Publishers.

Hardiman, Mariale. (2012). *The Brain Targeted Teaching Model*. Baltimore, MD: Johns Hopkins University.

Hunter, M. (1979, October). Teaching is decision making. *Educational Leadership*.

Hunter, M. (1982). *Mastery Teaching*. El Segundo, CA: TIP Publications.

Jensen, Eric. (2005). Teaching with the Brain in Mind—Applying Brain Research in Your School System. Association for Supervision and Curriculum Development, Virginia.

LeDoux J. E. (1994). Emotion, memory and the brain. *Scientific American 270*, 50–57.

LeDoux J. E. (1996). *The Emotional Brain*. New York: Simon & Schuster.

LeDoux, J. E. (2000). Emotion circuits in the brain. *Annual Review of Neuroscience 23* 155–184.

LeDoux, J. E. (2002). *Synaptic Self: How Our Brains Become Who We Are*. New York: Viking

Marzano, Robert. (2006). *Classroom Assessment and Grading That Work*. Alexandria, VA: Association for Supervision and Curriculum Development.

Marzano, R. J. (2007). *The Art and Science of Teaching: A Comprehensive Framework for Effective Instruction*. Alexandria, VA: Association for Supervision and Curriculum Development.

Marzano, R., Pickering, D., and Pollock, J. E. (2001). *Classroom Instruction That Works*. Alexandria, VA: Association for Supervision and Curriculum Development.

Schiller, Pam, and Willis, Clarissa A. (2008, July). Using brain-based teaching strategies to create supportive early childhood environments that address learning standards. *Young Children*.

Sousa, David. (2000). *How the Brain Learns*. Thousand Oaks, CA: Corwin Press.

Sousa, David. (2001). *How the Brain Learns* (2nd ed.). Thousand Oaks, CA: Corwin Press.

Sousa, David. (2001). *How the Special Needs Brain Learns*. Thousand Oaks, CA: Corwin Press.

Stape, Chris. (2009). Brain Research, Instructional Strategies, and E-Learning: Making the Connection.

Willingham, D. T. (2010). *Why don't students like school? In Why Don't Students Like School? A Cognitive Scientist Answers Questions About How the Mind Works and What It Means for the Classroom*. San Francisco: Jossey-Bass.

Wolfe, Pat. (1999). Revisiting effective teaching. *Educational Leadership*, 56(3).

Appendix A
Classroom Environment

Classroom Environment

Teacher: _____ Room: _____ Grade: _____ Date: _____

	Rubrics	Meaningful feedback	Routines and labeling	Student Work Posted
Highly Effective	- Rubrics and exemplars are posted and used - When possible, students have contributed to the development of a rubric - Students refer to rubrics to monitor their progress – self regulate and self management of time and learning.	- Feedback is accurate and constructive - Feedback is specific - Feedback is provided in a timely manner - Students can apply the feedback for future learning -	- Routines are well established causing no loss of instructional time. - Routines are posted or evident and promotes self regulated learning. Instructional charts, - anchor charts and labels promote student directed learning. - Smooth transitions	- Student work is current - Posted work consists of creative student projects - Student work can serve as exemplars of high student expectations - Student work shows pride, attention to detail and rigor
Effective	- Rubrics are posted, infrequently used. - Students are encouraged to monitor their work – Self Regulate their learning - Students use the rubrics for Self Regulated Learning (SRL) - Exemplars posted	- Feedback is accurate - Feedback varies on papers from specific to global - Feedback is provided in a timely manner and for all the papers posted.	- Routines or procedures posted to ensure smooth transitions and effective use of instructional time - Routines are posted or evident and stress high expectations for students - Students transition from one activity to the next smoothly.	- Student work posted varies from high to moderate rigor - Student work current but limited in scope - Posted work consists mainly of student projects with no worksheets -
Partially Effective	- Some rubrics are posted - Students are aware of the criteria for a specific project or task - Students are aware of the rubric and self monitor or assess	- Feedback is limited and for one subject - Feedback is generic on some papers and not on other papers - Feedback is provided in a timely manner for most of the papers -	- Routines do not appear evident causing loss of instructional time. - Routines are posted or evident by ineffectively applied. - Routines or procedures are posted for class behavior	- Some student work posted - Posted student work has current and non current examples - Posted work a mix of worksheets and student projects -
Ineffective	- Rubrics are not posted - Students are not aware of the criteria for grading - Students do not engage in self assessment	- Feedback is very limited and sporadic - Feedback is generic for all papers. Global comments are used "very good" - Feedback is not provided in a timely manner	- Routines do not appear evident causing loss of instructional time. - Routines are not posted or evident - Students are confused by a lack of routines or procedures	- Minimal student work posted - Student work is not current - Posted work consists mainly of worksheets -
Student Questions	- *What is the purpose of the rubrics?* - *How often do you use the rubrics?*	- *Does the teacher's feedback challenge you?* - *How does the teacher's feedback help you learn?*	- *Do you know what to do when you are finished with your assignment?* - *How were the routines established?*	- *Why is their student work posted?* - *What do you do if your work is not posted?*

Classroom Environment

	Student Work	Meaning feedback	Routines and Labeling	Rubrics
Ratings Highly Effective	- Current - Creative - Serve as exemplars	- Accurate - Specific - Timely - Can be applied for future learning	- No loss of instructional time - Posted - Smooth transitions	- Posted - Developed by students - Used by students
Effective	- Posted with high to moderate rigor - Work current but limited - Student projects displayed	- Accurate - Feedback varies - Timely for many students	- Posted and stress high expectations - Smooth transitions most of the time - Some labeling	- Posted, infrequently used - Students encouraged to use - Some SRL
Partially Effective	- Some student work posted - Work not current - Mostly worksheets	- Limited and sporadic - Generic or global comments - Not timely	- Routine not evident or posted - Loss of instructional time - Lack of routines	- Some rubrics are posted - Students are aware of the criteria - Limited use of rubrics
Ineffective	- Minimal work posted - Work two months or longer or older - Posted work mostly worksheets	- Limited and sporadic - Mostly global comments - Feedback not timely.	- Not evident - Loss of instructional time - Students confused by lack of structure	- Not posted - Students not aware of rubrics - No student self assessment

Appendix B
Differentiating Instruction

Teacher: _____ **Room:** _____ **Grade:** _____ **Date:** _____

	Ineffective	Partially Effective	Effective	Highly Effective
Content	- Lesson not tied to standards, does not engage the student, lacks rigor. Only recall-and-remember types of questions - Assessment does not guide instruction. - Content not tied to real-life or applicable - Lesson not tiered - No self regulation used - No relationship of student objective to essential question	- Lesson tied to standards but lacks rigor. Low levels of questioning to promote application - Sporadic assessments or monitoring of less content - A reference made to application of content but focus is on acquiring facts - Occasional grouping used - Very limited self-regulation	- Lesson tied to standards, some rigor for selected students, application promoted - Assessments used to assess lesson but does not cause lesson to be adjusted based on the information gained - Occasional reference to application of material and use - Groups are static or fixed - Infrequent self-regulation	- Lesson has rigor and requires higher levels of thinking, tied to standards - Frequent checks for understanding employed - Assessments used to monitor and adjust the lesson - Flexible grouping used - Students self-regulate during the lesson
Process	- Teacher does not incorporate student learning styles - Strategies promote factual recall or low level of knowledge use - No adjustment in rate of instruction or opportunity to practice skills - Large group instruction	- One learning style predominately used - Strategies promote the application of declarative knowledge - Limited or infrequent monitoring of lesson to determine effectiveness. - Large group instruction with limited small groups	- Two different learning styles used on a limited basis - Strategies promote development of procedural knowledge skills of analysis or evaluation - Frequent monitoring of lesson with adjustments made and opportunities provided to practice the skill - Small groups used but all students working on same task	- Variety of learning styles used throughout the lesson - Strategies promote meta-cognition - Adjustment of lesson made based on feedback and opportunities to practice provided - Variety of instructional strategies used based student needs
Product	- Summative assessment used - Assessment criteria not clear or posted for student. - No variety for student assessments and only one skill at a time assessed, usually at end of lesson	- Limited or infrequent use of formative assessments - Assessment criteria posted but not used by student. - One form of assessment used, i.e., paper/pencil and/or based on criteria other than standards, eg., neatness or effort	- Frequent use of formative assessments - Assessment criteria posted and available to student - Assessment based on a limited selection or group project but does not involve student choice or selection	- Formative and summative used - Assessment material posted and used for student to self-regulate - Variety of assessments used based on student choice and tied to the use of standards

	Ineffective	Partially Effective	Effective	Highly Effective
Interest	- No grouping of students - No connections of material to student interest - Student interest identified - Student product and outcomes same for whole class with teacher example provided	- Limited grouping of students, based on skill not interest - Material connected to real world but not interest - Limited and/or infrequent connection to student interest - Outcomes broad based with some exceptions	- Some flexible grouping based on interests - Material connected to some student's interests - Some connection of material to student interest - Product or outcomes based on selected pre-determined examples provided by teacher	- Grouping of students by interest and are flexible - Material connected to student interest - Promote interest beyond classroom - Student suggests choice of project or centers - Products based on student interest and varied use of MI
Readiness	- Expectation is all students have prerequisite skills - Instruction focused on "average" with no differentiation for student abilities or readiness - No grouping	- Limited assessment of skills as groups are fixed - Some modification made to curriculum or instruction - A small group of students occasionally used	- Occasional assessing of students for grouping - Curriculum modified based on student needs and some groups developed according to ability - Some flexible grouping based on student skill level	- Assessments determine grouping - Curriculum modified based on student levels - Flexible grouping used based on student interest and abilities

Dispositions "Look fors"	Ineffective	Partially Effective	Effective	Highly Effective
Content "Look fors" Standards based, inter-disciplinary, rigorous, student centered, authentic	- Large group instruction used - Lack of relationship between lesson and application of discipline. Recall of facts promoted - Limited application of use of material	- Limited use of any small group instruction - Lesson linked to standards but a low level of rigor - Content focused on knowledge and understanding of material	- Large group introduction followed by small group instruction - Content focused on analysis and application of material (low levels of questions leading to high levels of application or high level of questions and activities)	- Tiered activities - Independent activities - Interdisciplinary lesson with higher levels of application - Problem-based learning promoted to show deep understanding of concepts and application
Process "Look fors" Structured, dynamic, monitored, and adjusted based on feedback, promotes Self-Regulated Learning (SRL)	- Lesson lacks a clear structure with routines not apparent. A "filler for the period" - Students wait for teacher to move ahead - No mini-strategies or lesson adjustment used to differentiate instruction based on individual response or CFU - All students have same assessments and will produce the same product to show mastery	- Lesson has a structure and "agenda" but not followed - Students, with teacher permission, can use an additional resource., - Lesson plan dictates student need not feedback from students - Some advanced students able to complete a different assessment or product	- Lesson has structure and agenda with smooth transitions between activities - Student must ask permission to use different or varied resources - Some strategies used to develop flexible groups, i.e., lesson compacting, tiered activities, feedback from DOL, CFU, assessments. - Students can work in groups to produce a product	- Students move at their own pace and self-manage their time. - Student can select from Anchor activities or other resources - Strategies in place to plan and execute compacting the lesson, i.e., student learning contracts, independent study, SRL - Students use multiple intelligences to produce product
Product "Look fors" Summative, diverse, MI used, shows what student knows	- One product used for all students - Product based on low-level interpretation of the skill or concept - No reference to world application	- Teacher-directed product for entire class - Product based on low-level interpretation with mid-level production, i.e., application - A reference to real-world application	- Teachers provide product and student can make some modification to the product - Product requires higher level of interpretation, i.e., evaluation or creation - Some reference to real-world connections	- Based on student application of information using analysis, interpretation, or creativity - Use of multiple intelligences for product based on student ability - Real-world application

Dispositions "Look fors"	Ineffective	Partially Effective	Effective	Highly Effective
Interest **Student involvement activities, student connections, self-regulation**	- Low level of student participation, lesson teacher directed - Activities same for all students - Students compliant but not self-regulating - No connection of material to interest	- Large group instruction, teacher directed with some reference to interest - Limited activities planned or executed - Limited or infrequent connection of material to student interest	- Student involvement based on occasional reference to identified student interest - Occasional reference to student's interest or activities geared to individuals - Reference made to specific students	- Instruction based on student interest to promote student involvement - Activities student centered and based on individual interests - Specific and frequent reference to student interest
Readiness **Student skill levels, grouping, assessments to determine levels**	- Teacher expects all students to have prerequisite skills - Teacher pace same for all students - Learning environment doesn't promote SRL - Limited resources for student use.	- No pre-testing done and infrequent assessments to determine groupings - Teacher determines pacing and learning is lock-step - Resources available, posters, rubrics posted but not used	- Pre-testing done to determine grouping and assessments used to monitor progress - Varied pacing or students determine their pace, use environment to promote self-regulation	- Teacher uses assessments to determine grouping of students - Students engage in SRL, constitutionally and environmentally - Resources available and students encouraged to use them

Appendix C
Objective DSL Indicators

Teacher: _____ Room: _____ Grade: _____ Date: _____

Student Learning Target (Objective) and DSL(s) w/ Indicators

	Student Learning Target (Objective)	Demonstration of Student Learning (DSL)	Indicators
Highly Effective	- A procedure is in place and students look for the daily objective - Objective aligned Common Core - Objective aligned with CRT, curriculum benchmark, or curriculum map - Objective referred throughout lesson to promote self-regulated learning	- Clear connection to objective - High-level verbs used - Student friendly - Measurable–assesses what was taught - Multiple assessment measures can be used to show mastery - DSL tied to multiple pathways	- High-level verbs used - Objective and DSL linked and aligned to standards - Objective and DSL written in student friendly terms and appropriate for the age/grade level
Effective	- Objective an outcome and not an activity - Mid-level verbs used to promote cognition - Objective is clear, specific, and measureable - Content and process linked and lead to development of "dispositions"	- Assessment can be linked to other disciplines - DSL uses high level of Revised Bloom's Taxonomy - DSL will allow student to create other measures of assessment - DSLs will lead "dispositions"	- Objective and DSL is clear and specific - Objective and DSL are measurable - Students know what they are expected to learn and how they will be assessed - Objectives reflect "dispositions," for example, student will not only know how to read but will have a desire to read.
Partially effective	- No procedure is in place but teacher will tell student what the objective is for the day - Outcome is moderately clear - Verbs are mid-level on Bloom's Taxonomy (Apply and Application) - Objective is specific with low expectations for students - Objective and DSL are congruent with learning activities	- DSL posted and there is a connection to what is being taught. - Moderate level of rigor expected (Bloom's mid-level of the Taxonomy, such as apply and application) - DSL provides opportunity for integration with other disciplines	- Objective/DSL congruent - Objective/DSL address mid-level of Revised Bloom's Taxonomy - Students can articulate objective and DSL and see the relationship to other disciplines - Moderate rigor planned or assessed - Opportunity for interdisciplinary tasks - The objective and DSL are specific to the activities planned
Ineffective	- No objective listed - Objective not aligned to standards or curriculum map - Objective is an activity and not stated as a learning outcome - Objective does not permit skill acquisition - Objective uses verbs that promote low-level expectations with no application of skills - Planned activities not congruent with objective	- DSL not connected to objective - Students are not aware of how they will be assessed - Low-level verbs used for the assessment - Objective/DSL low level of rigor - No clear criteria for assessment - DSL not written in student friendly terms	- Objective not posted - An activity, not objective, is listed - Verbs used are Bloom's low level or knowledge and comprehension - Objective/activity does not suggest or allow for an assessment - Objective/DSL does not promote self-management or self-regulation - Student cannot articulate what they are expected to learn or how they will be assessed

	Student Learning Target (Objective)	Demonstration of Student Learning (DSL)	Indicators
Student Interview Questions	- What are you learning today? - Is what you are doing today going to help you learn today's objective? - Do you feel today's lesson has high expectations for your learning?	- How will you show the teacher what you learned today? - What are other ways to show the teacher you learned today's lesson?	- Students will show or can self-regulate and monitor their learning throughout the lesson - Students can self-regulate and monitor for the assessment

© M. Barbiere EdD, May 2012, updated March 2013, 2017. This rubric is copyrighted; permission to use must be obtained.

This rubric and other rubrics are in Dr. Barbiere's texts and Field Guides: *Teaching to the Learner's Brain and Activating the Learner's Brain*

Overall Rating: _____

Follow-up: ____ yes ____ no

Follow-up Date: _____

Notes:

_____

_____

_____

_____

_____

_____

_____

_____

Next Steps:

_____

_____

_____

_____

_____

Verbs used	
Congruence between objective and DSL	
Objective conveys high expectations	
Self-monitoring or self-management "I" statements used	
Outcomes are written using Revised Bloom's higher levels	
Other	

© M. Barbiere EdD, May 2012, updated March 2013, 2017. This rubric is copyrighted; permission to use must be obtained. This rubric and other rubrics are in Dr. Barbiere's texts and Field Guides: *Teaching to the Learner's Brain and Activating the Learner's Brain*.

Appendix D
Objective DSL Checklist

Checklist for development of Student Learning Target (Objective) and Demonstration of Student Learning (DSL)

	Objective		Indicators	Considerations/Tasks
Alignment	- Objective ties to Essential Question - Objective aligns with Common Core State Standards - Objective addresses a skill to be assessed by a CRT, curriculum benchmark or curriculum map - Aligns to district curriculum	☐ ☐ ☐ ☐	- High-level verbs used - Objective and DSL linked and aligned to standards - Objective is an expectation for skill development and not an activity	- Are Common Core standards "unpacked" in the development of the objective? - Does the objective lead to deeper understanding of the concept? - What is the desired student outcome?
Behavior	- Objective is written using "I" - Objective stresses a student outcome and is not an activity - Lower levels of Revised Bloom's Taxonomy (RBT) used to promote factual knowledge that will lead to application (developmental level of skill) or - Higher-level verbs used to promote metacognition - Content and process linked and leads to the development of "dispositions"	☐ ☐ ☐ ☐ ☐	- Begins with "I can, I will" - Clear, specific, measurable so students know what to do - RBT used to develop factual knowledge and base for developing application - Higher-level verbs used in the assessment of the skill - Is the skill needed for the development of a disposition?	- Objective and DSL written in student friendly terms and appropriate for the age/grade level to promote Self-Regulated Learning (SRL) - Factual knowledge necessary to develop creative thinking (Willingham, 2011) to develop skill base for later use - Assessment (DSL) requires analysis or evaluation to show mastery - "Disposition," for example, student learns how to read to develop a desire to read.
Condition	- Various strategies planned to deliver the lesson - Delivery of the lesson addresses various student modalities - Technology planned to enhance lesson - Delivery will promote varied grouping practices (large or small groups)	☐ ☐ ☐ ☐	- Instructional strategies used based on student needs - Variety of learning styles used throughout the lesson - Technology planned for teacher and student use - An outcome of the delivery will lead to flexible grouping	- Varied modalities planned throughout the year - Students will be able to work at their own pace and self-manage their time - Technology available for student use and differentiation of lesson - Flexible grouping or use of anchor activities for students who finish early
DSL/ Measurement	- Clear connection to objective - High level of Bloom's Taxonomy verbs used to assess the learning - Written in student friendly terms - Measurable–assesses what was taught - Multiple measures of assessment can be used to show mastery - Assessment can be linked to other disciplines - DSL will allow student to create other measures of assessment - DSLs will lead to "dispositions"	☐ ☐ ☐ ☐ ☐ ☐	- Objective/DSL congruent - RBT used with emphasis on analyze, evaluate, or create - Students can articulate DSL - Measurement based on rubric or standards - Opportunity for the use of some multiple intelligences - Interdisciplinary approach used for the activities planned - Student will be able to use multiple measures - DSL mastery can lead to broader use of skill	- Based on student application of information using analysis, interpretation, or creativity - "I can" or "I will show" the teacher - Measurement known to student so student can self-assess throughout lesson - Use of multiple intelligences for product based on student ability - Real-world application promoted to show application of disciplines - Student expands original assessment to develop other assessments - Broader applications are expected

	Objective		Indicators	Considerations/Tasks
Teacher questions	- What will the student be learning today? - How will I cognitively challenge the student? - Do I feel today's lesson has high expectations for their learning?	Student expectation	- Student products will reflect deeper understanding and application of skills - Students will think of other ways to show the teacher they learned today's lesson	- Students can self-regulate and monitor throughout the lesson as they know what they are learning and how they will be assessed - Students will use varied assessments to show teacher their depth of knowledge

© M. Barbiere, EdD, April 2013. May 2013 . This rubric is copyrighted; permission to use must be obtained.
This rubric and other rubrics are in Dr. Barbiere's text: *Setting the Stage: Teaching to the Learner's Brain*

Appendix E
Student Engagement

Teacher: _____ Room: _____ Grade: _____ Date: _____

	Student Engagement	Indicators
Highly Effective	- Activities are student directed and planned for student involvement - Students initiate or adapt activities or assignments - Materials and resources promote student engagement - Lesson has high degree of student involvement as teacher facilitates the lesson - Multiple instructional strategies used - A variety of learning styles are used in the delivery– auditory, visual, and tactile experiences are provided - Multiple-response strategies are employed - Students initiate choice, adaption, or creation of materials	- Students know what to do when they enter the room and begin to work independently - Cooperative activities are planned or group work is conducted; teacher facilitates the process - Multiple learning styles are used throughout the lesson - Students are able to self-regulate their learning either by self-management or self-monitoring - Multiple response strategies used - Teacher checks of understanding every 5–7 minutes and adjusts accordingly
Effective	- Activities vary from student directed to teacher directed - A majority of time devoted to student involvement - Materials and resources promote student engagement - Lesson has high degree of student involvement as teacher facilitates the lesson - Multiple instructional strategies used - A variety of learning styles are mostly used in the delivery; auditory, visual, and tactile experiences are provided - Multiple-response strategies are employed	- Students know what to do when they enter the room and begin to work independently - Cooperative activities are planned or group work is conducted. Teacher facilitates the process - Multiple learning styles are addressed sporadically throughout the lesson - Some students are able to self-regulate their learning either by self-management or self-monitoring - Multiple-response strategies used sporadically - Teacher checks of understanding every 8–10 minutes and adjusts accordingly
Partially Effective	- Activities are appropriate to some students - Materials and resources do not promote students - Lesson has sporadic student involvement but more teacher directed - There is marginal student involvement as most of the lesson is teacher driven - One learning style (auditory) is used during the lesson - Limited multiple responses–mostly choral responses	- Some activities are varied for students - There is some student activity as students are working - Two learning styles are used but most of the instruction is lecture - Some students will know what to do but most wait for the teacher to direct them - Teacher checks for understanding and uses one or two strategies
Ineffective	- Students come late, enter the room, and wait for the teacher to tell them what to do - Students are compliant but not intellectually engaged - Lesson is teacher driven - One learning style is used during the lesson (auditory) - Students not sure of what to do next, cannot regulate their own learning - No multiple-response strategies - Few checks for understanding	- Activities are teacher directed with minimal student involvement - Lecture-driven lesson with little student involvement - Students are compliant but not engaged - Students need to be told what to do or will frequently ask the teacher what to do next - Teacher has limited checking for understanding and continues lesson after a few students respond
Student Questions	- *What are you expected to do when you enter the class?* - *What do you do if you finish early?* - *What are your responsibilities for group work?*	- *Guiding Question: What are the students doing as a result of what the teacher has said or done?* - *Are the students cognitively challenged or compliant?* - *Can students manage and monitor their time effectively and independently?*

Overall Rating: _____

Follow-up: ____ yes ____ no

Follow-up Date: _____

Notes:
_____
_____
_____
_____
_____
_____
_____
_____
_____

Next Steps:
_____
_____
_____
_____
_____

Student Engagement "Look Fors"

Learning styles used	
Multiple response strategies used	
Checking for understanding	
Self monitoring or self management	
Independent learner	
Teacher facilitation	

Appendix F
Student Interviewing

Student Interviews

	What are you learning? (Forethought: Phase 1 of SRL, Wolter, 2010)	**How do you assess your learning?** Monitor Learning: Phase 2 Zimmermann,, 2000)	**Why studying?** Use, management and regulation of learning strategies: Phase 3	**When you need assistance?** Reflection: Final stage of SRL
Highly Effective	- Student explains learning in specific and concrete terms. - Student provides an analysis of the learning. - Students are aware of the criteria for a specific project or task. - Student describes the expected outcome.	- Students use the learning environment (exemplars, rubrics, posted work) to assess their learning - Students monitor their learning - Conduct a similar DOL as the one by the teacher—adapting activities	- Student evaluates the lesson and makes a real world connection - Student demonstrates self regulation strategies for the expansion of the lesson - Student relates the learning to goals (EQ or unit) and career	- Students identify others who can help them - Students seeks other sources for assistance - Students develop ways to self regulate - Students develop and use ways to self manage their time and work - SRL strategies used
Effective	- Student explains more than the lesson objective - Student explanation is clear and specific - Student makes connections to other disciplines - Student uses "I statements" or indicates self monitoring in another manner	- Teacher feedback used - Students are aware of the rubric for use to self monitor or assess - Peer review used - Written feedback from assignments used to promote learning - Multiple ways used, ie., teacher, student developed, district, to assess the learning	- Student able to make a connection to real world situations - Student can explain necessary milestones for the next grade or graduate - Student dispositions or habits of mind exhibited for higher level learning. - Student can apply the lesson to future learning	- Student knows three options before asking the teacher - Student frequently uses the classroom environment for assistance. - Student uses notes, work folders, journals to self regulate the learning.
Partially Effective	- Student states the learning objective only. - Student re-states objective using I" because if it written as such. No internalization	- Limited use of assessments by students - Student has a source for assessing their learning, in the room or personally, but is not used.	- Student occasionally self assess their learning to expand their learning. - Student occasionally contributes to class discussion	- Student will wait for the teacher to get help. - Student occasionally seeks help from another student. - Limited use of resources to get help
Ineffective	- Student can not state what they are learning. - Student does not have "ownership" (does not use I statement) of the objective . - No objective posted so student unaware of the expectation.	- Student not aware of any way to assess their learning. - Student does not use any source within the room to assess their learning. - Student does not have a source for assessing their learning, i.e., rubric.	- Student compliant and does not contribute to expansion of the learning during large group instruction. - Lack of student participation or willingness to contributions to discussion	- Student waits for teacher to answer questions or concerns. - No effort is made by student to get help from classmate or classroom environment. - Student prefers to have teacher explanation.
Student Questions	- *What are you learning today?* - *How will you learn?* - *How is what your learning important?*	- *Are you accomplishing your work?* - *How do you know you are doing well?* - *What questions do you ask yourself when you study?*	- *How will you plan to complete the assignment?* - *How does this assignment relate to the final product?*	- *Why do you seek help from your peers?* - *Can you resubmit your assignments? If so, how do you use the feedback you received from your first submission when you revise your work?*

Appendix G
Use of Data

Use of Data to Inform Instruction

Teacher: _____ Room: _____ Grade: _____ Date: _____

	Rubrics	**Meaningful feedback**	**DSLs/Formative Assessments**	**Student Self Regulation**
Highly Effective	- Rubrics and exemplars are posted and used - When possible, students have contributed to the development of a rubric - Students refer to rubrics to monitor their progress – self regulate and self management of time and learning.	- Feedback is accurate and constructive - Feedback is specific - Feedback is provided in a timely manner - Students can apply the feedback for future learning	- Frequents checks for understanding to monitor and adjust the learning. - Multiple measures used. - Feedback from assessment is used to guide instruction - Do Now differentiated - DSLs conducted individually, or in small groups	- Students are actively engaged in assessing their own learning - Students use the learning environment to assess their learning - Student assessments used for improvement as evidenced by re-submissions - Students help each other
Effective	- Rubrics are posted, infrequently used. - Students are encouraged to monitor their work – self regulate their learning - Students use the rubrics for Self Regulated Learning (SRL) - Exemplars posted	- Feedback is accurate - Feedback varies on papers from specific to global - Feedback is provided in a timely manner.	- Moderate checking for understanding via choral responses. - Feedback given from the formative assessments is sporadically applied to guide instruction. - Data from the Do Now is used for instruction - DSL planned but not conducted	- Students assess their learning to determine corrections, modifications or adjustments. - Students use environment to promote learning - Students aware of criteria and use rubrics
Partially Effective	- Some rubrics are posted - Students are aware of the criteria for a specific project or task - Students are aware of the rubric and self monitor or assess	- Feedback is limited and for one subject - Feedback is generic on some papers and not on other papers - Feedback is provided in a timely manner for most of the papers -	- Limited or infrequent checking for understanding (CFU) - Data collected but not used - Feedback from a few students directs the flow of the class - Do Now/DSL/Closure not differentiated	- Students do not engage in self regulation unless the teacher directs or prompts them. - Classroom management procedures curtail the ability of students to engage in self regulation.
Ineffective	- Rubrics are not posted - Students are not aware of the criteria for grading - Students do not engage in self assessment	- Feedback is very limited and sporadic - Feedback is generic for all papers. Global comments are used such as "very good" - Feedback is not provided in a timely manner	- No monitoring of student work via checks for understanding or formative assessments - Teacher directed lesson with no feedback sought - No DSL conducted - No Do Now	- Students are teacher directed and not student directed - Students do not self regulate
Student Questions	- *What is the purpose of the rubrics?* - *How often do you use the rubrics?*	- *Does the teacher's feedback challenge you?* - *How does the teacher's feedback help you learn?*	- *How does the teacher know if you know the material?* - *How do assessments help guide your learning?*	- *What do you do if you have a problem with the assignment?* - *How manage your time?*

Use of Data to Inform Instruction

SRL – Self Regulated	Metacognition	Procedural	Conceptual	Factual Knowledge
	Rubrics	Meaningful feedback	Assessments	Self Regulation
Highly Effective	<ul><li>Posted</li><li>Developed by students</li><li>Used by students</li></ul>	<ul><li>Accurate</li><li>Specific</li><li>Timely</li><li>Can be applied for future learning</li></ul>	<ul><li>Frequent CFUs or assessments conducted</li><li>Assessment data drives instruction</li><li>DSLs conducted</li><li>Do Now is varied</li></ul>	<ul><li>Environment established to promote SRL</li><li>Student monitoring done</li><li>Student manages time and work</li></ul>
Effective	<ul><li>Posted, infrequently used</li><li>Students encouraged to use</li><li>Some SRL</li></ul>	<ul><li>Accurate</li><li>Feedback varies</li><li>Timely for many students</li></ul>	<ul><li>Checks for Understanding (CFU) sporadic</li><li>Limited ways of CFU</li><li>Lesson marginally adjusted as a result of the CFU or assessment</li></ul>	<ul><li>Work posted reflects student revisions</li><li>Students assess their learning</li><li>Student projects displayed</li></ul>
Partially Effective	<ul><li>Some rubrics are posted</li><li>Students are aware of the criteria</li><li>Limited use of rubrics</li></ul>	<ul><li>Limited and sporadic</li><li>Generic or global comments</li><li>Not timely</li></ul>	<ul><li>Limited CFU</li><li>Limited assessments used</li><li>Instructional time not impacted by assessments</li></ul>	<ul><li>Some student work posted</li><li>Work not current or useful for SRL</li><li>Mostly worksheets used</li><li>SRL strategies infrequently mentioned</li></ul>
Ineffective	<ul><li>Not posted</li><li>Students not aware of rubrics</li><li>No student self assessment</li></ul>	<ul><li>Limited and sporadic</li><li>Mostly global comments</li><li>Feedback not timely.</li></ul>	<ul><li>CFU not done</li><li>Instructional time not impacted by CFU</li><li>Assessments not done or planned</li></ul>	<ul><li>Minimal work posted thereby not promoting SRL</li><li>Work two months or longer or older thereby not useful for SRL</li><li>SRL strategies not promoted</li></ul>

About the Author

Dr. Mario C. Barbiere has administrative experience at all district levels, as well as college (associate professor) and State of New Jersey level. He has extensive experience in school turnaround, beginning with serving as network turnaround officer for two inner-city schools in New Jersey that had been low performing. Working with the principal and teachers, both schools doubled their test scores in one year and became higher-achieving schools.

Following that, Dr. Barbiere was executive director for Regional Achievement Center, Region 5, created to work with low-performing schools or schools with an achievement gap. Under the Every Student Succeeds Act (ESSA), the Regional Achievement Centers were identified as Comprehensive Support and Improvement (CSI) teams, and Dr. Barbiere served as the regional executive director for CSI 3, covering seven counties in New Jersey.

Dr. Barbiere's doctoral studies were in brain research and lesson design. The research developed interest in instructional delivery and student self-regulation.

Having the opportunity to work in a variety of schools, Dr. Barbiere is passionate about teaching and student empowerment so students are empowered and self-dependent not teacher or school dependent.

www.ingramcontent.com/pod-product-compliance
Lightning Source LLC
Chambersburg PA
CBHW081831300426
44116CB00014B/2546